Jules Korby

Great Ormond Street
and the Story of Medicine

by
Jules Kosky
and
Raymond J. Lunnon

Published by The Hospitals for Sick Children, London,
in association with Granta Editions.

© J. Kosky and R. J. Lunnon and The Board of Governors of The Hospitals for Sick Children

First published 1991

ISBN 0 906782 61 9

Published by The Hospitals for Sick Children, London,
in association with Granta Editions, 47 Norfolk Street, Cambridge CB1 2LE

Granta Editions is an imprint of The Book Concern Ltd

British Library Cataloguing in Publication Data
Kosky, Jules
  Great Ormond Street and the story of medicine.
  I. Title   II. Lunnon, Raymond J.
  362.19892000942142
  ISBN 0-906782-61-9

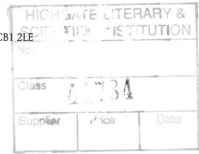

ACKNOWLEDGEMENTS

The authors wish to thank the following without whose assistance the publication of this book would not have been possible: the Special Trustees of The Hospitals for Sick Children for their support and encouragement to publish this book and also that of Mr John Quinton, formerly Director of the Fundraising Department; Dr A. P. Norman, for many years a senior member of the medical staff of the hospital, for his careful reading of the text, his suggestions, comments and advice; the Department of Medical Illustration, The Hospitals for Sick Children and Institute of Child Health, Director, Simon E. Brown and his staff for their professional help with the photography of many items; the Wellcome Institute Library, London, and Mr William Schupbach and Mr David Brady for their considerable help enabling the publication of Figs. 10, 20, 22, 24, 30, 31, 32, 34, 35, 37, 38, 51, 62 and 63; Dickens House and Dr D. Parker for permission to use Figs. 7, 15 and 19; the Children's Hospital of Philadelphia and Miss Shirley Bonnem, Vice-President for permission to publish Figs. 12 and 27; the Marie Curie Foundation for Fig. 68; the Audiovisual Department of the National Hospital for Neurology and Neurosurgery and Institute of Neurology (Director, George Kaim) for permission to use Figs. 70 and 71; the Audiovisual Department of St Mary's Hospital, Paddington (Director, Emrys Sparks) for permission to use Figs. 93 and 94; the Education and Medical Illustration Service, St Bartholomew's Hospital and Medical School (Director, Professor P. G. Cull) for permission to use Fig. 101; Norwich Health Authority for permission to use Fig. 23 from their publication *Jenny Lind in Norwich* by S. M. Bishop, J. S. Buist and M. J. Flynn; the Coram Foundation for permission to reproduce Figs. 5 and 117; the parents of the patient shown in Fig. 107 for permission to publish this photograph of their daughter; Powell, Moya and Partners for providing photographs and illustrations of the redevelopment of the hospital, Figs. 111, 112, 113 and 121;

the Oxford University Press for permission to quote from Sir Peter Medawar's *Pluto's Republic* (1982) and to reproduce Fig. 109 from *Inborn Errors of Metabolism*, A. E. Garrod (1909); the Royal College of Physicians for permission to reproduce Figs. 3 and 110; Fig. 21 is reproduced from *Friedrich-Wilhelms-Universitat zu Bonn*, Henry and Cohen, Bonn (1839); Figs. 66, 77, 100 and 104 are reproduced from an article on The Hospital for Sick Children in *The Sphere*, No. 1137 dated November 5th, 1921; Fig. 28 is based on an original in the British Museum; Fig. 79 is reproduced from *Barrie: The Story of a Genius*, by J. A. Hammerton, Sampson Low (1929); Fig. 116 is reproduced from a lithograph entitled *Florence Nightingale at Scutari*, published by Paul and Dominic Colnaghi, dated 21st April 1856.

Other illustrations are from the photographic libraries of the Museum and Archives and the Department of Medical Illustration, The Hospitals for Sick Children.

Every effort has been made to obtain permission for the reproduction of the illustrations and extracts in this book; apologies are offered to anyone whom it has not been possible to contact.

The authors are also indebted to:
Mrs Jean Carroll of the Fund Raising Department, The Hospitals for Sick Children, for her considerable help, encouragement and advice; Nicholas Baldwin, Fellow Archivist at The Hospitals for Sick Children for his help; Miss Tammie Fisher, of the Fundraising Department of The Hospitals for Sick Children, for typing the original manuscripts; Miss Elaine Brooke, Librarian, Institute of Child Health, for her assistance with access to the West Library. We would also like to acknowledge the co-operation given by the staff of Book Connections Ltd, Cambridge.

Design and production in association with Book Connections, Cambridge.

Typeset by Anglia Photoset, Colchester.

Printed and bound by Proost N.V., Turnhout, Belgium.

Contents

This book is dedicated to the
Children, Parents and Staff of
The Hospitals for Sick Children, London,
and
Children's Hospitals Everywhere.

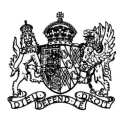

KENSINGTON PALACE

This book, written and produced on behalf of The Hospital for Sick Children in Great Ormond Street, tells how this great hospital has developed since its modest beginnings in 1852. The story of medicine is also told from its ancient beginnings to the present day and further anticipates even more impressive advances in the future.

Every parent whose child has had to be admitted to hospital knows what a worrying time this can be and this book will help generate a broad understanding of the development of paediatric medicine and child care now practised in many parts of the United Kingdom and elsewhere in the world.

As President of The Hospital for Sick Children, I am very happy to commend it not only to parents and guardians but also to all those of any age, who have an interest in the welfare of children in the past, present and future.

Diana.

September, 1991

A Table of the First Children's Hospitals up to 1900

Including Some Early Dispensaries, Infirmaries and Clinics for Children

1769 LONDON: Dr George Armstrong's Dispensary for the Infant Poor (the first dispensary for children in Europe; it closed in 1781)

1787 VIENNA: Dr J. J. Mastalier's Children's Dispensary

1802 PARIS: Hôpital des Enfants Malades (the first children's hospital in Europe)

1810 BRÜNN (BRNO): Dr Ringolini's Children's Dispensary

1816 LONDON: Dr John Bunnell Davis's Universal Dispensary for Children

1820 LONDON: Royal Western Infirmary for Children (dispensary only)

1821 DUBLIN: The National, a children's clinic

1829 MANCHESTER: General Dispensary for Children

1834 ST PETERSBURG: The Nicholas Children's Hospital
BERLIN: Children's Clinic at the Charité
DRESDEN: Children's Clinic

1837 VIENNA: Dr Mauthner's Children's Hospital

1839 BUDAPEST: Children's Clinic

1840 HAMBURG: Children's Hospital
LONDON: Kensington Dispensary for Children

1842 MOSCOW: Children's Hospital
FRANKFURT: Children's Hospital
VIENNA: St Joseph's Children's Hospital
PRAGUE: Kaiser Franz Joseph Children's Hospital
STUTTGART: Children's Hospital

1843 BERLIN: Elizabeth Children's Hospital

1844 BERLIN: Louisa Children's Hospital
GRAZ: Children's Hospital

1845 BUDAPEST: Children's Hospital
LEMBERG (LVOV): Children's Hospital
COPENHAGEN: Children's Hospital
TURIN: Children's Hospital (for girls only)
STOCKHOLM: Children's Clinic

1846 BRÜNN (BRNO): Children's Hospital
MUNICH: Children's Hospital

1847 CONSTANTINOPLE: Children's Hospital

1851 STETTIN: Children's Hospital
LIVERPOOL: Institution for Diseases of Children (clinic)

1852 LONDON: The Hospital for Sick Children, Great Ormond Street (the first children's hospital in the United Kingdom)

1853 NORWICH: Jenny Lind Children's Hospital

1854 STOCKHOLM: Crown Princess Louisa Children's Hospital
PARIS: Sainte Eugénie Children's Hospital

1855 MANCHESTER: Children's Hospital
LEIPZIG: C. Hennig's Polyclinic and Children's Hospital
PHILADELPHIA: Children's Hospital (the first children's hospital in America)

1857 LIVERPOOL: Children's Hospital
BRISTOL: Children's Dispensary
LEEDS: Children's Hospital

1860 EDINBURGH: Royal Hospital for Children

1862 BIRMINGHAM: Children's Hospital
NEWCASTLE: Children's Hospital
BASLE: Children's Hospital
BERNE: Jenner Hospital for Children

1863 LONDON: Belgrave Children's Hospital

1864 SUNDERLAND: Children's Hospital

1865 AMSTERDAM: Emma Hospital for Children
CHICAGO: Mary Thompson Children's Hospital

1866 LONDON: Grosvenor Children's Hospital
Victoria Hospital for Children, Chelsea

1867 LONDON: Queen Elizabeth Hospital for Children,
          Bethnal Green (originally the North-
          Eastern Hospital for Children)
      GLOUCESTER: Children's Hospital
      LONDON: Alexandra Hip Hospital, Queen Square

1868 LONDON: East London Hospital for Children,
          Shadwell
      BRIGHTON: Children's Hospital
      ZURICH: Children's Hospital

1869 LONDON: Evelina Children's Hospital
      NOTTINGHAM: Children's Hospital
      BIRKENHEAD: Children's Hospital
      BOSTON: Children's Hospital

1870 MELBOURNE: Children's Hospital
      NEW YORK: St Mary's Children's Hospital

1871 WASHINGTON, DC: Children's Hospital

1872 LONDON: Sydenham Road Children's Hospital
      HULL: Children's Hospital
      SEVENOAKS: Children's Hospital
      DUBLIN: Children's Hospital
      BELFAST: Ulster Children's Hospital

1873 ATLANTIC CITY: Children's Hospital
      RADNOR, Pa: Children's Hospital

1874 LONDON: Cheyne Children's Hospital, Chelsea
      CHELTENHAM: Children's Hospital
      CORK: Victoria Children's Hospital

1875 TORONTO: Hospital for Sick Children
      LE HAVRE: Children's Hospital
      ALBANY, NY: Children's Hospital
      SAN FRANCISCO: Children's Hospital

1876 SHEFFIELD: Children's Hospital
      BOMBAY: Children's Hospital
      ADELAIDE: Children's Hospital
      CRACOW: Children's Hospital

1877 BRISBANE: Children's Hospital

1878 DRESDEN: Children's Hospital

1879 HELSINKI: Children's Hospital
      ST LOUIS: Children's Hospital

1881 CREMONA: Children's Hospital
      NAPLES: Lina Children's Hospital
      BOSTON: Infant's Hospital

1882 MADRID: Infant Jesus Children's Hospital

1883 LONDON: Paddington Green Children's Hospital
      BRADFORD: Children's Hospital
      GLASGOW: Royal Glasgow Hospital for Children
      OPORTO: Maria Pia Children's Hospital

1884 BALTIMORE: Thomas Wilson Sanitarium for
          Children
      CHICAGO: Children's Memorial Hospital

1885 BRISTOL: Children's Hospital

1886 NEWBURY: Children's Hospital
      NEW YORK: Laura Franklin Hospital for Children

1887 GATESHEAD: Children's Hospital
      DETROIT: Children's Hospital
      NEW YORK: Babies' Hospital
      SYRACUSE, NY: Children's Hospital

1888 TORQUAY: Rosehill Children's Hospital

1890 GENOA: Children's Hospital

1892 MILWAUKEE: Children's Hospital
      BUFFALO: Children's Hospital
      COLUMBUS, OHIO: Children's Hospital

1893 LONDON: St Mary's Hospital for Children, Plaistow

1897 ABERDEEN: Royal Hospital for Children

1899 LIVERPOOL: Royal Liverpool Country Hospital for
          Children

1900 ATHENS: St Sophia Children's Hospital
      NANCY: J. B. Thierry Children's Hospital
      PARIS: Bretonneau Children's Hospital
          Trousseau Children's Hospital
          Pasteur Children's Hospital

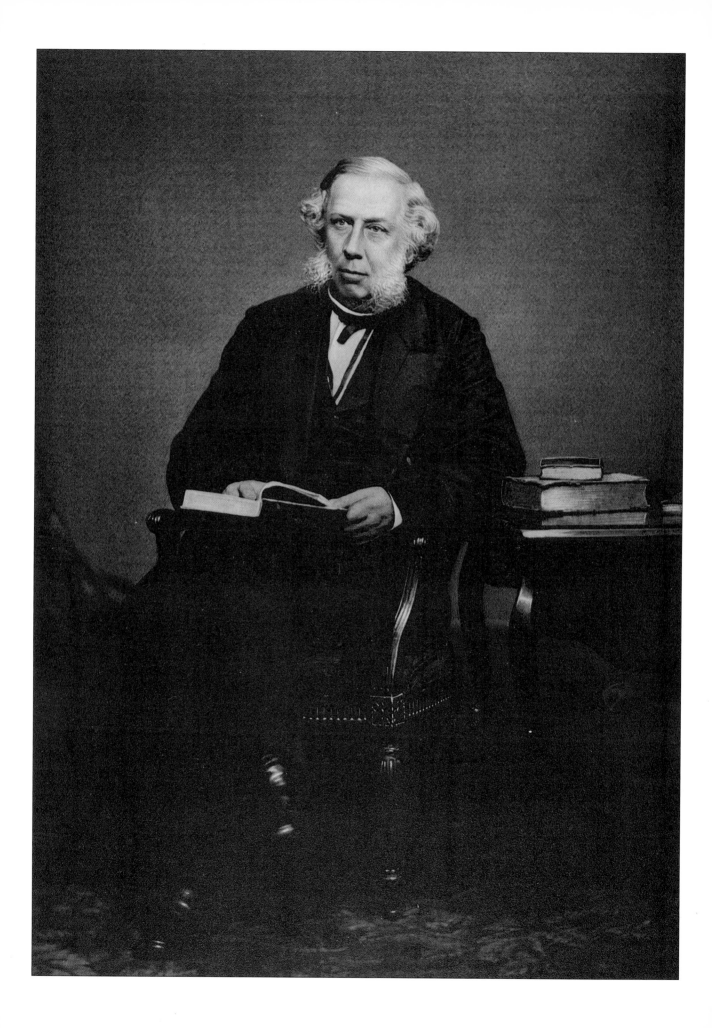

CHAPTER 1

Introduction

Why Great Ormond Street began

The Hospital for Sick Children, Great Ormond Street, opened in February 1852. It was largely the inspiration and effort of one man: Dr Charles West. Children's hospitals, as distinct from the earlier foundling hospitals and orphanages, had existed in Europe since Paris set an example in 1802, but Great Ormond Street was the first children's hospital in the United Kingdom. As Dr West's original *Appeal to the Public in Behalf of a Hospital for Sick Children* pointed out in 1850, neither in London 'nor throughout the whole British Empire is there any hospital exclusively devoted to their reception'. A few children's dispensaries or infirmaries were scattered around the country, but these only accepted children as out-patients, giving mothers such advice and medicines as were then available. Dispensaries and hospitals for women, mostly lying-in or maternity hospitals, treated babies and sometimes infants, but on a very limited scale.

The great teaching hospitals of the time usually restricted their advice on children's diseases to a few paragraphs at the end of a standard course of lectures on women's diseases and midwifery. This made Dr West decide to give his first series of lectures in 1847 on the *Diseases of Infants and Children* at the Middlesex Hospital.

A few children, mostly the victims of accidents or those needing surgery, were admitted to general hospitals, where they lacked the necessary special attention and nursing. For a few years Guy's Hospital had a small children's ward with thirteen beds in a wooden building over some old stables. The London Hospital had an accident ward with seventeen beds for children under the age of 7. It was no wonder that in January 1843, of the 2,363 patients in all the London hospitals, only 136 were children under 10, and only 26 of these children were suffering from an internal disease and were not accident or surgical cases. Yet nearly half of the 50,000 people who then died every year in London were children. As Dr West commented bitterly, children's diseases were little studied and poorly understood. He knew that only a children's hospital could remedy the situation.

From its modest beginnings with only ten beds, Great Ormond Street has become the world's most celebrated children's hospital. Its story is of interest to children and parents everywhere: not only do its patients come from all over the UK but also from all over the world. Its fascinating history runs side by side with an equally important story, the advance of modern medicine. The story of one will help to explain and encourage interest in the other, especially among children. And Great Ormond Street's story will also be in many ways the story and celebration of other children's hospitals, many of which were inspired and shaped by its example. To understand its own special spirit and tradition is to understand the spirit of love and concern that exists in children's hospitals everywhere.

There are still too many children suffering from deprivation and disease today: they are always the first to be struck by famine and disaster, in open warfare or civil conflict. But, though much still remains to be done in large parts of the world, children today are more fortunate than those of the past. Many of the infectious diseases and fevers which once harrowed them are now virtually eliminated. Millions are no longer crippled by poliomyelitis. Girls know that when they become mothers their chances of dying in childbirth, or shortly afterwards from puerperal fever, are slight compared to sixty years ago. Surgery has ceased to be an agonising and perilous horror; its recent advanced techniques have given adults and children, and now even the unborn, the gift of a continued full and active life.

Children have also benefited from social progress, from special legislation, from improvements in public health, hygiene and nutrition, and from a growing concern for their welfare, environment and education. Paediatrics today deals with the total well-being of children, from new-born babies to adolescents, as well as with their specific illnesses and physical or organic defects. Dr West's understanding of this came from visiting his young patients at home and seeing the terrible conditions 'sunk in squalid poverty' in which they lived. In his first appeal for a children's hospital, he expressed his belief that it would become 'a means of moral as well as of physical good, and another link in the golden chain of benevolence and gratitude which should bind together all classes of society'.

The Hospital for Sick Children's neighbouring and co-operating Institute of Child Health – founded in 1946 in collaboration with the University of London, the Ministry of Health, and

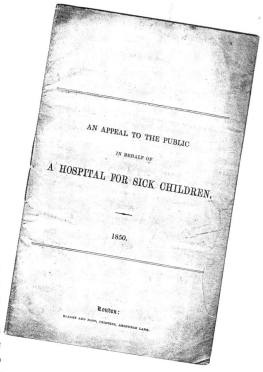

2 The appeal leaflet published in 1850 to stimulate interest in and raise funds for the establishment of a children's hospital in London.

LEFT: *1 Dr Charles West, MD (1816–98), founder of The Hospital for Sick Children.*

London County Council – is the modern expression and development of Dr West's hopes. Its programme of research and international instruction also confirms another of his prophecies when he argued that such a hospital would benefit not only the children of the poor but those of all classes, because of the improvements in the knowledge and treatment of their diseases it would bring. In fact, the whole of humanity has gained: many of the great advances in medicine first involved and concerned children. The story of Great Ormond Street, like that of other children's hospitals, shows us that over the last 150 years there have been few more valuable contributions to the welfare and future of mankind.

A history of children's medicine

The treatment and care of sick children only became a specialised branch of medicine as paediatrics in the middle of the nineteenth century, when modern medicine began and Great Ormond Street opened. Little had been written before then on children's diseases; what there was dealt mostly with childbirth and infant rearing. The general view since antiquity had been that the care of children was best left to their mothers and nurses. Until the time of Dr West, the average doctor knew little about childhood illnesses although he may have been reasonably skilled in obstetrics, the procedures before, during and after birth. In Charles Dickens's words they could do no more than 'shake their heads with vain regret over the little corpse, around which women weep so bitterly'. A shocking example of this ignorance is found in some statistics from Sweden where, in the middle of the eighteenth century, 9,783 of all the children that died in one year were recorded as dying 'from unknown causes'. At that time the total population of Sweden was a little over 1,700,000.

The first doctor whose name we know was Imhotep of Egypt, who lived around 2700 BC. The earliest medical texts were also Egyptian. One of these, the Ebers Papyrus of 1500 BC, gave remedies for childish complaints, distinguishing between children and adults in drugs and dosages. Imhotep was deified and became associated with Asklepios, the Greek god of medicine. Hippocrates, born in 470 BC, was the greatest doctor in Greece and indeed in antiquity; the famous Hippocratic Oath is still taken by doctors today. Free from superstition, Hippocrates was medicine's first scientific observer. He noted how children reacted more quickly than adults to disease (something Dr West always impressed upon his pupils and nurses), how they were more likely to die from wounds and could not tolerate fasting. His medical theory of the Four Humours that needed to be balanced in the body dominated medical thought for two thousand years.

Towards the end of the reign of the Roman Emperor Tiberius, around AD 30, Cornelius Celsus wrote *De re Medicina*, the earliest Latin medical work. It was the first to state firmly that 'children require to be treated entirely differently from adults'. But one hundred years were to pass before Soranus of Ephesus wrote *On Diseases of Women*, part of which is the first ever study of children's diseases. He dealt with the care of mothers, the rearing of babies and some of the more common childhood diseases. It set a pattern. But there was no real advance in obstetrics until the sixteenth century, and nearly everything written on children's diseases after Soranus, even until the eighteenth century, was based on him, sometimes almost repeating him word for word.

The Islamic doctors who advanced the study of medicine between the tenth and twelfth centuries in Persia and Moorish Spain eagerly translated Soranus together with Hippocrates and the great Graeco-Roman doctor Galen, including them in their own vast encyclopaedic medical writings. Rhazes the Persian was the first to distinguish between measles and smallpox, a landmark in medical history. Translated in its turn into Latin, Arabic medicine thus passed the almost forgotten medical lore of Greece and Rome back to Europe.

But despite the recovery of these classical texts, the opening of medical schools and universities, the founding of hospitals, of retreats for lepers and of asylums for abandoned children, European medicine deteriorated. During the Middle Ages poor sanitation, dirt and ignorance of hygiene led to epidemics and plagues. In some areas, the Black Death of the fourteenth century wiped out more than a quarter of the population. If children survived the perils of being born – as late as the sixteenth century even the wealthiest households made little attempt at cleanliness during labour or afterwards – they were left to the care of mothers and nurses who used the old folklore medicine of charms and simple herbal remedies. Perhaps, like the poor, they were much the better for it. The rich, after being bled and purged almost to death by their surgeons and physicians, swallowed weird, nauseating, complicated, expensive but mostly useless concoctions prepared by apothecaries. If they did not die of the disease, they died of the cure!

Not until the sixteenth and seventeenth centuries with Vesalius's work on anatomy, Galileo's experiments and Harvey's discovery of the circulation of the blood, were science and medicine freed from a blind acceptance of Aristotle's and Galen's authority. Children's diseases, however, still had to wait for another century before receiving proper attention.

The invention of printing

On the invention of printing, one of the earliest medical books and the first treatise on paediatrics to be published was Bagellardo's *Libellus de Egritudinibus* at Padua in 1472. A German work on children's diseases, the first to be published in the vernacular, appeared a year later at Augsburg: Metlinger's *Ein Regiment der Jungen Kinder*. Both these works, after five centuries, were still based on the Persian doctors, Rhazes and Avicenna, sometimes quoting them almost word for word and repeating much of what Soranus had written in the second century AD.

The first work to be written in English on children's diseases was *The Boke of Children* printed in London in 1545. The author, Thomas Phaer, who came from Cardigan, is better remembered as a poet and an early translator of Virgil's *Aeneid*. Again, much of the subject matter is based on the old Greek, Roman and Arabic authorities. Later in the sixteenth century, Guillaume de Baillou became dean of the medical faculty at the university of his native Paris. He died in 1616, but his works were published posthumously in 1640. His *Epidemiorum* gave the first detailed account of whooping cough. Although the disease was already known – in England it was popularly called chin-cough – no medical writer had previously dealt with it. Baillou described an epidemic of whooping cough in 1578 which 'attacked children of four months, ten months, and a little older, and carried off an enormous number ... The lung is so irritated that ... the patient seems to swell up, and as if on the verge of suffocation ... The paroxysm of coughing repeats, sometimes so distressing that blood is driven out by its violence, through nose and mouth.'

The first detailed description of rickets as a definite disease of the softening of children's bones was written by an English doctor, Daniel Whistler. It was his doctoral thesis at Leyden University, and was published there in 1645, ten years before the famous work on the same subject by Francis Glisson. In 1660 Samuel Pepys met Dr Whistler, describing him in his diary as 'good company and a very ingenious man'.

Thomas Sydenham (1624–89) was one of the greatest doctors in history. He is looked upon as the founder of modern clinical medicine and was called the 'English Hippocrates'. He was the first to describe chorea, or St Vitus' Dance, a nervous disorder afflicting children from about the age of 10, which causes involuntary movements of the limbs and face and general muscular weakness. The name 'Sydenham's Chorea' is still used. Sydenham also wrote the most detailed and careful description of measles that had yet appeared, and his report on scarlet fever was the first under that name.

Sydenham's friend, the famous philosopher John Locke, who had studied medicine at Oxford, published *On Education* in 1693. This, together with works published earlier in the century by Comenius in Germany and Sweden and Sir William Petty in London, marked a new approach to the care and education of children of all classes, and a better understanding of their needs and place in society. It was to be the start of a movement towards social justice and an awakening of the social conscience that led, among other reforms, to the founding of special children's hospitals in

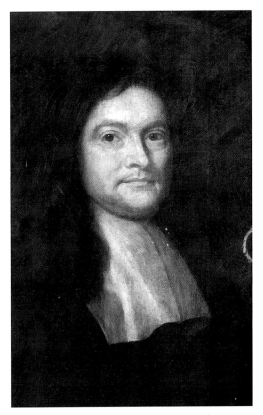

3 Dr Daniel Whistler c. 1641–84.

Europe and eventually to that at Great Ormond Street.

Thomas Sydenham is said to have inspired and given his patronage to the best seventeenth-century book on children's diseases: the *Acute Diseases of Infancy*, which Walter Harris, physician to Charles II and William of Orange, had printed in London in 1689. This was the year of the Bill of Rights, which finally established constitutional monarchy and guaranteed the freedom of the English Parliament. With excessive modesty Sydenham told Harris: 'Your little book may be of more service to the public than all my own writings.' Harris's 'little book' was reprinted many times in its original Latin and in its English translation and appeared in French, German and other versions. For a hundred years it remained the first in its field in England until supplanted in 1784 by Michael Underwood's *The Diseases of Children*. And Underwood's book itself remained in use until Dr West published his own *Lectures on the Diseases of Infancy and Childhood* in 1848.

TIME CHART

BC
c. 2700 Imhotep of Egypt, the first doctor named in history.
c. 1500 Ebers Papyrus, the first medical manuscript.
c. 470–c. 400 Hippocrates, the Greek father of medicine.
384–322 Aristotle, the codifier and founder of science.

AD
c. 30 A. Cornelius Celsus: *De re Medicina*. The first medical treatise in Latin.
c. 130 Soranus of Ephesus: *On Diseases of Women*. Contains the first treatise on children's diseases.
199 Galen of Pergamon, the great Graeco-Roman physician whose authority remained almost undisputed until the sixteenth century, dies.
c. 829 Hôtel Dieu Hospital at Paris first mentioned.
c. 850 The medical school at Salerno founded.
c. 923 Rhazes, the great Persian physician, dies.
980–1037 Avicenna, the Persian physician whose *Canon* was the most famous medieval encyclopaedia of medicine.
1080 A hospital for lepers opened near Canterbury.
1110 University of Paris founded.
1120–1200 Medicine flourishes in Moorish Spain with Avenzoar, Averroes and Maimonides.
1137 St Bartholomew's Hospital, London, founded.

1140 Medical school at Bologna.
1167 University of Oxford founded.
1209 University of Cambridge founded.
1347–8 Black Death in England and Europe.
1472 Bagellardo: *Libellus de Egritudinibus*. The first printed book on the diseases of children.
1543 Andreas Vesalius: *The Fabric of the Human Body*. The beginning of modern anatomy.
1545 Thomas Phaer: *The Boke of Children*. First book written in English on children's diseases.
1564–1642 Galileo. The beginning of modern science.
1628 William Harvey: *De motu cordis*. The circulation of the blood.
1640 Guillaume de Baillou: *Epidemiorum*, published posthumously. The first detailed account of whooping cough.
1645 Daniel Whistler first describes rickets.
1654 Francis Glisson describes rickets more fully.
1665 The Great Plague of London.
1686 Thomas Sydenham, the English Hippocrates, describes chorea.
1687 Sir Isaac Newton: *Principia Mathematica*. The greatest of all scientific works and perhaps the supreme achievement of the human intellect.
1689 Walter Harris: *Acute Diseases of Infancy*.
1693 John Locke: *On Education*.

CHAPTER 2

The Olden Days

Rosen van Rosenstein

Paediatric medicine began with the publication in 1765 of Nils Rosen van Rosenstein's *The Diseases of Children and their Remedies*, in Stockholm, where Rosenstein was physician to the King of Sweden. Appalled at his colleagues' ignorance of children's diseases, as revealed by the contemporary bills of mortality, Rosenstein was instrumental in obtaining a royal mandate ordering the Stockholm Lying-in Hospital to launch the first series of lectures on the diseases of infancy in 1761. Sir George Frederic Still, the first doctor at Great Ormond Street to confine his work only to children even outside the hospital, wrote nearly two centuries later that Rosenstein and Michael Underwood stood out as the most scientific and illuminating of all the writers on children's diseases in the eighteenth century. In 1784, Underwood gave the first account of poliomyelitis, and in 1799 an early account of congenital heart disease in children.

Rosenstein's book differs from most of its predecessors in only once mentioning an ancient writer. He refers to contemporary books, scientific societies and his own case-notes. He was ahead of his time in advising that children's food should be covered so that 'no insect or any such thing can get at it'; if feeding bottles had to be used, they should be kept scrupulously clean. Long before Pasteur, Rosenstein came close to the idea of bacterial infection when describing whooping cough: 'The true cause of this disease must be some heterogeneous matter or seed, which has multiplicative power, as is the case with smallpox. Whether this multiplicative miasma be a kind of insect I cannot affirm with certainty.'

Dr West had read Rosenstein's work. In his library, now preserved at Great Ormond Street, is a copy of the Italian translation printed in 1780. Dr West also owned copies of Michael Underwood's and George Armstrong's treatises. But there were other influences in the eighteenth century which shaped, pioneered and nurtured his devotion to the cause of children's hospitals.

Christianity and Islam had early in their histories forbidden infanticide and the abandoning of unwanted babies – something that was rife in Greek and Roman civilisation and among primitive tribes – but the cruel custom continued. In the same way, laws and edicts against child slavery were ignored, even in modern times. Datheus, Archbishop of Milan, founded the first asylum for abandoned infants in AD 787. His example was followed throughout Europe in succeeding centuries; similar institutions were opened in Baghdad, Cairo and other places in the Moslem Empire. In France, of the foundling hospitals inspired by St Vincent de Paul, the patron saint of orphans, the most celebrated was the Hospice des Enfants Trouvés, in Paris, which Louis XIV chartered and endowed in 1670.

Squalor and death

Although orphanages, poor-houses and schools, such as Christ's Hospital, had long existed in England, the most famous was the London Foundling Hospital opened by Captain Coram in 1741 (see page 67). It is said that Coram was moved to found his institution by the sight of abandoned babies and young children left dead or dying on dung heaps in London streets. Two thousand years had made little difference to their fate – the same horrific sight had been seen in Hellenised Alexandria in the third century BC.

The mortality rates at these foundling hospitals became outrageously high: the worst example was in Dublin, where, of 10,272 infants received between 1775 and 1796, only 45 survived. In Paris, of 31,951 infants admitted between 1771 and 1777, 25,476 were dead before their first birthday. At Captain Coram's Foundling Hospital, of the first 15,000 children admitted, only 4,400 lived to grow up. Such grim figures, and the alarming mortality among infants and children farmed out to wet-nurses and foster-parents, were frequently quoted as an argument against hospitals for sick children. To Dr West, however, they were reasons in support of children's hospitals: he knew that without them, no progress could ever be made in the fight against the all-too-often fatal childhood ailments.

The first dispensary for children was opened on 24 April 1769 by George Armstrong at Red Lion Square, Holborn: something that had not existed before in England or, in fact, Europe. Within less than a century, the Hospital for Sick Children would open in Great Ormond Street, a few hundred yards from where George Armstrong's Dispensary for the Infant Poor had first functioned. Pioneer as he was, Dr Armstrong never believed that such a hospital would ever be possible. As he wrote in his account of the dispensary, although several supporters had thought a children's hospital should be considered, 'such a scheme

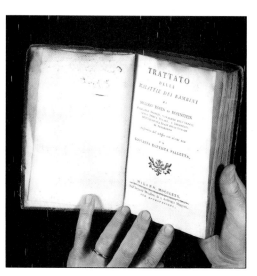

4 Dr West's own copy of an Italian edition of Rosen van Rosenstein's book on diseases of children.

can never be executed. If you take away a sick child from its parent or nurse you break its heart immediately.' A mother or a nurse to each child would so crowd the wards that 'the air of the hospital would be thereby much contaminated'. He emphasised the danger of infection spreading rapidly from one child to another.

The Dispensary for the Infant Poor lasted only a dozen years, after which lack of financial support and Dr Armstrong's own illness forced it to close. Like many pioneers, Dr Armstrong was little appreciated and died in obscurity. When the Universal Dispensary for Children, the first in England since Dr Armstrong's Dispensary, opened in 1816, its founder, John Bunnell Davis, confessed he had never heard of Dr Armstrong.

An immediate successor to Dr Armstrong lived in Vienna: Dr Mastalier opened a children's dispensary there in 1787. At about the same time a report was published on the squalid accommodation and unhygienic conditions at the Hôtel Dieu, the oldest general hospital in Paris, which can be traced back to the seventh century. There, sick children were crammed eight or nine together in one bed; nearly all of them died. Reform was constantly urged, but it was not until after the French Revolution that an orphanage in Paris was converted into the Hôpital des Enfants Malades in 1802. This was the first children's hospital to be opened anywhere in the world. The Hospital for Sick Children in Great Ormond Street echoed its name exactly fifty years later. George Armstrong's complaint, made in 1784, that too many doctors still thought it safer to entrust children 'to the care of old women', was at last being addressed.

Charles West

Charles West was born in London on 8 August in 1816, the year Davis started the Universal Dispensary for Children. The institution was to play a large role in Dr West's career. When Davis moved his dispensary to larger premises in Waterloo Road, in 1824, changing its name to the Royal Universal Infirmary for Children, two wards were actually planned for in-patients. But

Davis died a few months before the new building was opened, and, lacking his vision and enthusiasm, the Universal Infirmary ran into financial difficulties and the wards remained empty.

After serving an apprenticeship with an apothecary at Amersham, Charles West became a student at St Bartholomew's Hospital, London. He completed his training abroad, first at the University of Bonn, then in Paris, finally obtaining his doctor's degree in Berlin in 1837. Dr West had decided to specialise in women's diseases and midwifery, to which children's diseases at that time formed a complementary study. In Paris, the example of the Hôpital des Enfants Malades, still at that time almost the only hospital of its kind in Europe, had aroused his personal interest in, and sympathy with, sick children. It was certainly a strong factor in his later determination to open a London children's hospital. He first became officially associated with the Universal Infirmary for Children, Waterloo Road, in 1839, becoming its physician in 1842.

Dr West was also a physician at the Finsbury Dispensary, so he had in his charge children and, at Finsbury, their mothers from two of the poorest and most notorious slums in London. At the Finsbury Dispensary Dr West ministered to the very children Charles Dickens described so forcibly, quoting from his own *Oliver Twist*, at the Field Lane Ragged School, which he visited in 1843. Dr West's own case-notes on the children from that district add a grim, factual footnote to Dickens's eloquent picture of their appalling plight. Such a child was 10-year-old Anne Leach, who lived only a few yards from Saffron Hill. Her parents belonged, in West's own words, 'to that class of poor who seldom pay much attention to their children's ailments. When brought to me she was greatly emaciated.' Anne died six months after first coming under Dr West's care.

It was his work at Waterloo Road that gave Dr West unique knowledge and experience of children's diseases. As the famous surgeon Sir James Paget, his friend, fellow-student and colleague, was to remember many years later, 'Dr West worked among the sick poor in their own homes, with an enthusiasm unmatched, moved as he was both by his love of knowledge and by his pity for the sick poor. His pity could never be

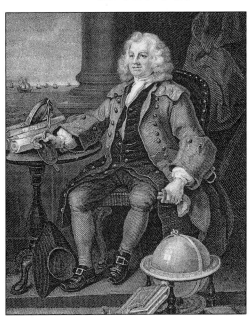

5 *Captain Thomas Coram, founder of the Foundling Hospital.*

satisfied.' He saw children like George Cole, aged 5, who suffered from endocarditis, an inflammation of the heart usually caused by rheumatic fever to which children were particularly susceptible. Dr West was able to save him. But 7-year-old Eliza Trewell, whom West recorded as 'the child of drunken parents living in the most squalid poverty', died of meningitis, in agony.

As Dr West knew, cities all over Europe, even in far Russia and Turkey,

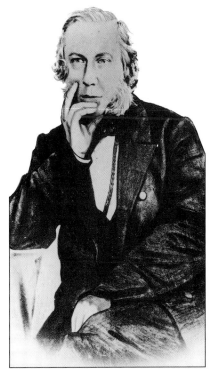

6 *Dr Charles West as a young man.*

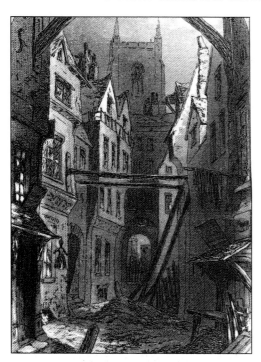

7 A Victorian illustration of 'Tom-all-alone's' from Bleak House showing the slum conditions which Charles Dickens knew so well, giving reality to his books.

were taking Paris as a model and opening children's hospitals. A favourite anecdote of his was how children recently discharged from the newly opened hospital at Frankfurt would gather outside the gates, pleading to be allowed to play in its garden again. Only in England, the richest country of all, were the sick children of the poor neglected by both private charity and government. From 1845 Dr West had pressed repeatedly for the still-unused wards at Waterloo Road to be opened and the Universal Infirmary turned into a true children's hospital. But the committee procrastinated and, as Dr West said, 'The attempt failed owing to the jealousies of local medical men.'

Dr West's professional reputation had grown over the years with the publication of his lectures given at Middlesex Hospital, and his appointment as lecturer at St Bartholomew's. In 1849 he resigned from Waterloo Road, determined to open a children's hospital elsewhere by his own efforts. He wrote to and visited leading London physicians and children's hospitals abroad, seeking information and active support. He received much sympathy and advice, but no practical assistance until one of the most famous doctors of the day, Richard Bright (whose name is remembered in kidney disease), suggested he approach

Dr Henry Bence Jones. Dr Bence Jones's wife was a daughter of the Earl of Gosford, and her sisters were interested in the idea of a children's hospital. Dr West and Dr Bence Jones met, quickly agreeing on plans to promote a hospital for sick children.

Dr West never forgot it was Dr Bence Jones who made his dream of a children's hospital possible; he remembered that debt thirty years later:

Dr Bence Jones had influential friends out of the profession, while I had none. The meetings of the Provisional Committee were held at his house; many persons, whom I had no means of approaching, were induced by him to join it, and but for his aid, the establishment of the Children's Hospital would have encountered far more difficulties than attended it: the attempt might even altogether have failed.

Bence Jones's influential friends included Lady Byron, the poet's widow, and her daughter, the Countess of Lovelace; the Earl of Shaftesbury, the great reformer and champion of defenceless children, who became chairman of the provisional committee and then the first president of Great Ormond Street; Baroness Burdett-Coutts, the richest

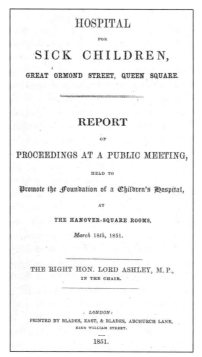

8 Report of a public meeting held to promote the foundation of a children's hospital, 18 March 1851.

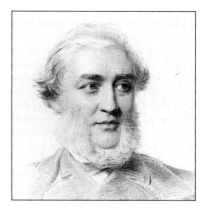

9 Dr Henry Bence Jones (1813–73), a principal supporter of the concept of a children's hospital.

woman in England and a famous philanthropist; the Earl of Carlisle and the Bishop of London. Charles Dickens was associated with them in many schemes of reform. Dickens's brother-in-law, Henry Austin, and friends, Dr Southwood Smith and Edwin Chadwick, all on the Board of Health, suggested and approved the necessary alterations to No. 49, Great Ormond Street.

Dr Bence Jones and Dr West were also successful in obtaining the vital support of many eminent doctors. This was later illustrated by a historic if sad episode in Victorian medicine. When Prince Albert died unexpectedly from typhoid nine years after Great Ormond Street opened, the four doctors attending him were Dr William Jenner, Sir James Clark, Sir Henry Holland and Dr Thomas Watson. The last three had supported Dr Bence Jones and Dr West from the beginning. Dr Jenner and Dr West were the first physicians appointed to Great Ormond Street.

Dickens to the rescue

The Hospital for Sick Children opened its doors on St Valentine's Day 1852 and was ready to receive patients two days later. But as Dr West reported, 'At first, indeed, it seemed almost as if a Children's Hospital was not needed.' During the first month only twenty-four children came to the out-patients, and only eight were received as in-patients. Six weeks after the hospital opened, however, Charles Dickens published 'Drooping Buds', the first description of the Hospital for Sick Children.

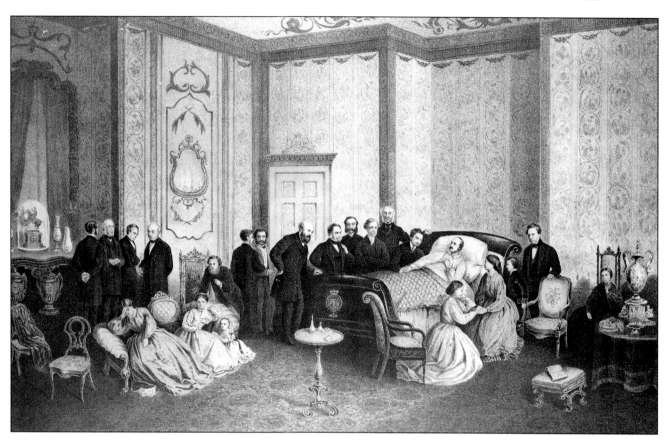

10 Death of HRH Prince Albert, 14 December 1861. A lithograph by H. L. Walton. Four physicians stand in an isolated group on the left. They are Dr William Jenner, Sir James Clark, Sir Henry Holland and Dr Thomas Watson. All had supported the concept of a children's hospital and Dr William Jenner was a physician to the Hospital for Sick Children at its inception.

The effect was immediate. Mothers came hurrying to Great Ormond Street with their sick children; they now knew and believed, in Dr West's own words, 'that those who asked for the suffering little ones were indeed to be trusted with so precious a deposit': a statement that sums up the history and meaning of Great Ormond Street, and is as true today as it was then.

A few weeks after 'Drooping Buds' appeared, Queen Victoria became the hospital's patron. Dickens's article prompted Norwich to open the Jenny Lind Children's Hospital in 1853 with money raised by the great singer. Dr West called it Great Ormond Street's 'first born'. Other children's hospitals soon opened in Liverpool and Manchester. Later, Dr West suggested that the reason why these two had overtaken Great Ormond Street in redevelopment was that Lancashire folk filled up cheques for their hospitals 'with three

"*Familiar in their Mouths as* HOUSEHOLD WORDS."—SHAKESPEARE

HOUSEHOLD WORDS.

•A WEEKLY JOURNAL•

CONDUCTED BY CHARLES DICKENS.

Nᵒ· 106.]   SATURDAY, APRIL 3, 1852.

DROOPING BUDS.

IN Paris, Berlin, Turin, Frankfort, Brussels, and Munich ; in Hamburgh, St. Petersburgh, Moscow, Vienna, Prague, Pesth, Copenhagen, Stuttgard, Grätz, Brünn, Lemberg, and Constantinople ; there are hospitals for sick children. There was not one in all England until the other day.

No hospital for sick children ! Does the public know what is implied in this ? Those little graves two or three feet long, which are so plentiful in our churchyards and our cemeteries—to which, from home, in absence from the pleasures of society, the thoughts of many a young mother sadly wander—does the public know that we dig too many of them ? Of this great city of London—which, until a few weeks ago, contained no hospital wherein to treat and study the diseases of children—more than a third of the whole population perishes in infancy and childhood. Twenty-four in a hundred die, during the two first years of life ; and, during the next eight years, eleven die out of the remaining seventy-six.

Our children perish out of our homes : not because there is in them an inherent dangerous sickness (except in the few cases where they are born of parents who communicate to children heritable maladies), but because there is, in respect of their tender lives, a want of sanitary discipline and a want of medical knowledge. What should we say of a rose-tree in which one bud out of every three dropped to the soil dead ? We should not say that it was natural to roses ; neither

gain more than cent. in the ten children.

It does not a gent physician successfully the i to modify his pla proportions of his of his knowled daughters. Som to themselves ; all, take a form from their fai varies from a or ought to b child's mind, an adult ; so act success ailments of thing, also attends o we are il and of taught, part of wail ; whe ans al

figures instead of two'. London gentlemen should follow this habit, or simply, 'sign their names and hand the blank cheque to the ladies to fill up!'

In 1853 an American physician, Dr Francis W. Lewis, visited Dr West in London and, inspired by his example, returned home to open the Children's Hospital of Philadelphia in 1855, the first in North America. So in effect all the great children's hospitals there sprang from the seed first planted by Dr West. The original ten beds at Great Ormond Street soon increased to thirty-

11   Charles Dickens wrote this article in Household Words *just six weeks after the hospital opened.*

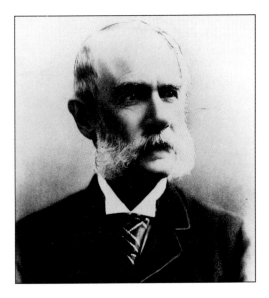

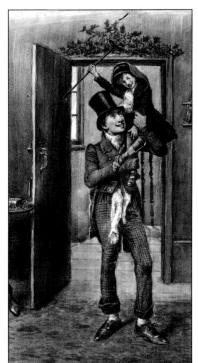

ABOVE: *12 Dr Francis West Lewis (1825–1902) of Philadelphia visited Great Ormond Street Hospital in 1853.*

ABOVE RIGHT: *13 Some of Charles West's own case-notes. In his time these were handwritten and patients' records were bound into large volumes under each doctor's name.*

one; by 1855 the number of out-patients had increased over six-fold from the first year's total of 1,250 to 8,087, and two assistant physicians were appointed. The Crimean War was at its height, and Florence Nightingale was at Scutari, laying the foundations of modern nursing (see page 67). In 1854 Dr West had anticipated her *Notes on Nursing* by five years with his *How to Nurse Sick Children*. It was a book with charm and authority which, he claimed, was 'written by a person who has seen a great deal of little children, especially of little sick children, who loves them very much'. Dr West had published it for the benefit of the hospital and his preface urged, 'Do not then let the Hospital fail for want of funds.'

This was a real danger in 1857, when the economic depression following the Crimean War reduced the hospital's capital to under £1,000.

Once more Dickens came to the rescue. The great novelist was also a great public speaker; to quote Anthony Trollope, Dickens 'had another gift – had it so wonderfully, that it might be said he has left no equal behind'. In 1858 Dickens appealed for funds at the Hospital Anniversary Dinner. It was the finest speech he ever made. Dr West remembered: 'Charles Dickens, the children's friend, first fairly set her [the Hospital] on her legs and helped her to run alone, and in a few eloquent words which none who have heard can ever forget. Like the good fairy in the tale, he gave her the gift that she should win love and favour everywhere; and so she grew and prospered.'

15 Tiny Tim in A Christmas Carol *by Charles Dickens.*

Dickens himself wrote: 'It is a good and kind charity. I hope and trust that I have happily been able to give it a good thrust onward into a great course.' His hopes were realised. Two months after making the speech, he read *A Christmas Carol* in aid of the hospital. His speech and reading raised nearly £3,000: enough to buy the house next door for £1,600 and double the number of beds. The hospital never looked back.

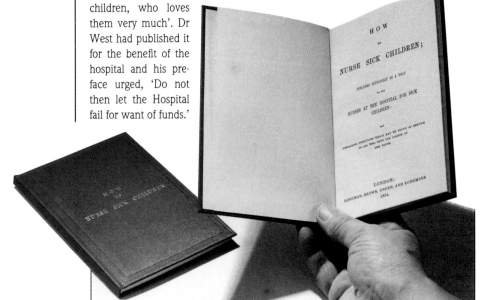

14 In 1854, Dr Charles West published his handbook for nurses entitled How to Nurse Sick Children, *intended as a help to the nurses at the Hospital for Sick Children.*

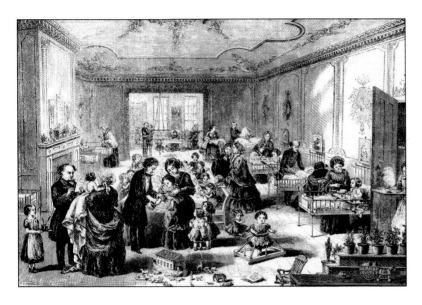

16 *An engraving dated 1858 which shows a ward in No. 49, Great Ormond Street, in which the two physicians are making their ward round – Dr Charles West (R) and Dr William Jenner (L). Notable aspects of this picture include parents attending their children, toys and a swing, the 'baby walker' and Dr Jenner holding a paper marked 'Diet Sheet'.*

The new hospital

The next landmark in Great Ormond Street's story was the building of an entirely new hospital, which would realise West's original dream of a chil-

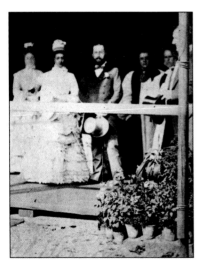

17 *The Prince and Princess of Wales at No. 49, Great Ormond Street, on 11 July 1872 on the occasion of the stone-laying for the new hospital building.*

dren's hospital with at least a hundred beds. The appeal for this was opened by Edward, Prince of Wales, at a hospital dinner in May 1870. This set a royal precedent that was followed by the Duke of Windsor when Prince of Wales, and then by Prince Charles for the Wishing Well Appeal. The foundation stone for the new building was laid by Alexandra, Princess of Wales, in 1872, and this precedent was followed by Diana, Prin-

cess of Wales, in 1991. The new building, designed by Edward Barry, 'furnished with every modern appliance for the alleviation of infantile diseases and sufferings', and with room for over a hundred beds, was opened in 1875 (see pages 64–5). More than fulfilling Charles West's prophecy that it 'will resound to the patter of little feet, and to the tinkle of tiny voices ... a hundred years to come', it was demolished only in 1990. The Hospital Chapel of St Christopher, also designed by Barry and donated by his brother William as a memorial to his wife, has been carefully preserved (see page 66 and, for its new location, page 68). With its gilt decorations, stained glass windows, and marble columns like a tiny Byzantine cathedral, it is, as Oscar Wilde said, one of the most beautiful hospital chapels in London.

A landmark of a different sort also belongs to 1875, when Dr West retired. He was made vice-president and the first consulting physician. In accepting this honour, he said: 'The one dream of my life has been to see the Children's Hospital well established, and that done I do not know that there is anything left for me to wish for.'

TIME CHART

AD

787 Datheus, Archbishop of Milan, founds first asylum for abandoned infants.
1670 The orphanage Hospice des Enfants Trouvés, Paris, endowed by Louis XIV.
1741 Captain Coram founds London Foundling Hospital.
1765 Nils Rosen van Rosenstein: *The Diseases of Children and their Remedies.*
1784 Michael Underwood gives earliest account of poliomyelitis.
1787 Report on conditions at Hôtel Dieu and other hospitals in Paris.
1816 Charles West born.
1824 Universal Dispensary for Children moves to Waterloo Road. J. Bunnel Davies dies.
1833–5 Charles West studies at St Bartholomew's Hospital.
1835–7 Charles West studies abroad at Bonn and Paris, and then at Berlin, where he takes his doctorate.
1839 Charles West begins working at the Royal Universal Infirmary, Waterloo Road.
1842 Charles West appointed physician at Waterloo Road.
1843 Charles West physician at Finsbury Dispensary. Charles Dickens visits Field Lane Ragged School in that area.
1845–9 Charles West tries to turn the Universal Infirmary into a children's hospital with in-patients.
1847 Charles West lectures at the Middlesex Hospital on diseases of children and infants. The lectures are published the following year.

1848 Charles West appointed lecturer in midwifery at St Bartholomew's Hospital.
1849 Charles West resigns from the Universal Infirmary. Seeks support for a children's hospital.
1850 First meeting of a provisional committee for a hospital for sick children at Dr Bence Jones's house.
1851 First public meeting in support of a hospital for sick children. No. 49, Great Ormond Street, acquired.
1852 The Hospital for Sick Children opened. Dickens publishes 'Drooping Buds'. Queen Victoria becomes hospital patron.
1853 Dr Francis W. Lewis of Philadelphia visits Dr West and Great Ormond Street, and returns home to open the first children's hospital in America.
1854 Florence Nightingale goes to Crimea. Charles West publishes *How to Nurse Sick Children.*
1857 Great Ormond Street threatened with closure owing to financial crisis.
1858 Charles Dickens raises funds by speaking at a public dinner and by a reading of *A Christmas Carol.* The hospital enlarged by purchase of house next door.
1859 Florence Nightingale: *Notes on Nursing.*
1870 Edward, Prince of Wales, launches rebuilding appeal for Great Ormond Street.
1872 Alexandra, Princess of Wales, lays foundation stone of a new hospital building.
1875 New Great Ormond Street Hospital building opened. Dr Charles West retires, becoming the hospital's first consultant physician.

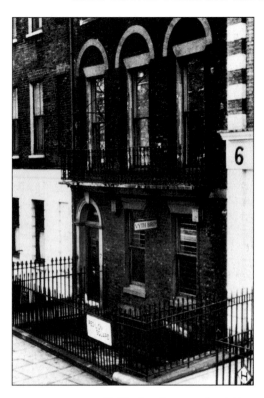

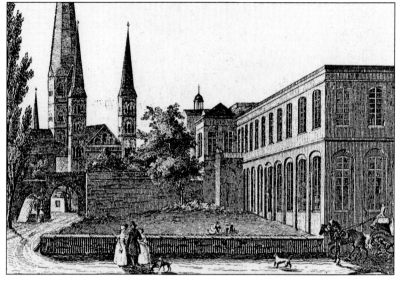

ABOVE: *21 The University of Bonn at about the time when Charles West was studying there.*

BELOW: *22 The Universal Dispensary for Children, Waterloo Road, London, established in 1816.*

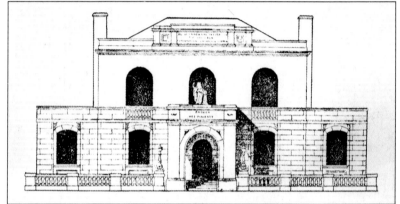

ABOVE: *18 The first dispensary for children was opened by Dr George Armstrong in 1769 in this house, No. 7, Red Lion Square, London.*

BELOW: *19 A photograph near Saffron Hill, probably taken in Edwardian times, showing the kind of gloomy slum areas which lay to the south and east of Great Ormond Street.*

BELOW RIGHT: *20 Vienna Children's Hospital (1837), the first of its kind in Austria.*

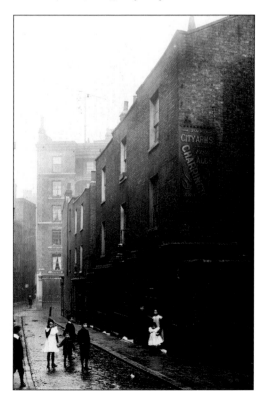

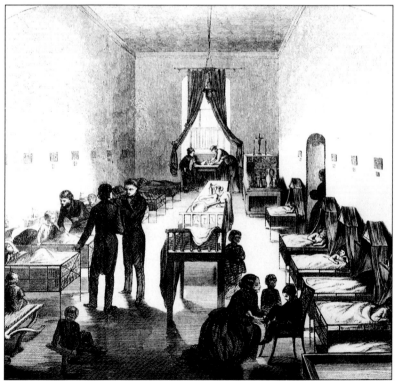

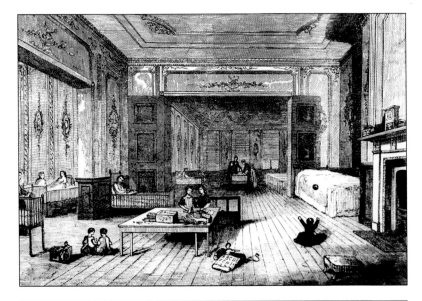

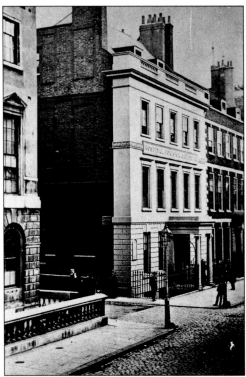

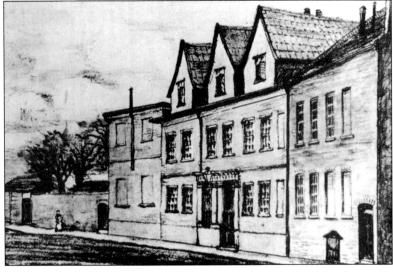

ABOVE: *25 The Hospital for Sick Children started in this house, No. 49, Great Ormond Street, in 1852.*

ABOVE LEFT: *26 The first engraving of a ward in the Hospital for Sick Children. Printed in 1852, the illustration shows some of the first patients admitted to the hospital.*

BELOW: *27 The original building of the Philadelphia Children's Hospital, which was the first in North America and was established in 1855.*

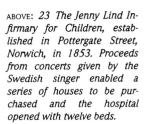

ABOVE: *23 The Jenny Lind Infirmary for Children, established in Pottergate Street, Norwich, in 1853. Proceeds from concerts given by the Swedish singer enabled a series of houses to be purchased and the hospital opened with twelve beds.*

RIGHT: *24 A sketch of the interior of No. 49, Great Ormond Street.*

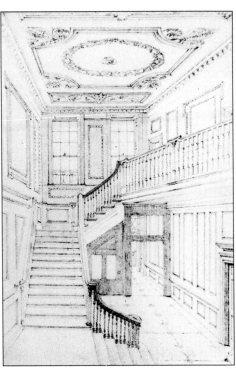

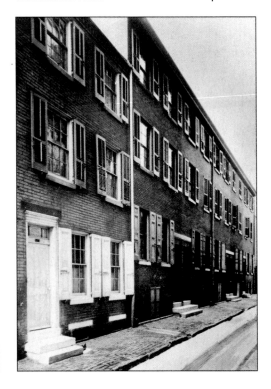

CHAPTER 3

The Bridge to Modern Medicine

Early strides

Dr West, like Sir William Jenner and most of the doctors and surgeons at Great Ormond Street in its early days, was a product of the British tradition of a medical apprenticeship followed by more training at the great teaching hospitals. Many years later, Dr West was to write of his apprentice days with nostalgia, of 'times and customs which for good or ill have passed away never to return'. But he, like many of his contemporaries, had also experienced the benefits of the Continental system, based mainly on those state-financed and controlled universities where scientific and medical research was centred.

The state of medicine around 1840, when Dr West began his professional career, was described by Sir Peter Medawar in 1972:

The physician of a hundred and thirty years ago was confronted by all manner of medical distress. He studied and tried to cure his patients with great human sympathy and understanding and highly developed clinical skills . . . The physician's relationship to his patient was a very personal one . . . But there was so little he could do! The microbial theory of infectious disease had not been formulated, viruses were not recognised, hormones were unheard of, vitamins undefined, physiology was rudimentary and biochemistry almost non-existent.

Dr West certainly had a large measure of sympathy and understanding with children. He had only to approach a crying baby in its mother's arms for the child to forget its tears, laugh, and hold out its hands to him. But the treatment at his disposal was very inadequate. By 1898, however, the year in which both Dr West and Dr Jenner died, the Curies had discovered radium, only three years after Röntgen first demonstrated the existence of X-rays; viruses were known to exist; and Ehrlich and others were beginning their crucial series of experiments on immunology, antibodies and chemotherapy.

Medicine made startling advances in the nineteenth century and within Dr West's lifetime for many reasons. The advances followed and went side by side with the scientist in his laboratory using instruments and equipment that were an outcome of the technology of the industrial revolution. Books such as Karl Friedrich Gauss's mathematical works in the early 1800s, Helmholtz's *Conservation of Energy* in 1847, and Darwin's *The Origin of Species* in 1859 were landmarks in scientific thought.

Historians suggest that the American and French Revolutions brought about not only a new intellectual and scientific renaissance, but also a growing social conscience, and a concern and legislation for public health and the protection of the poor and deprived, especially children. Certainly Edward Jenner, who discovered vaccination − 'one of the greatest triumphs in the history of medicine' according to the eminent medical historian F. H. Garrison − which was to save millions of children from an early death, did most of his work at that very time of political upheaval.

No. 49, Great Ormond Street had once been Dr Richard Mead's house. The spacious room he built to hold his famous library became the hospital's first out-patients department. Dr Mead, physician to Queen Anne and Sir Isaac Newton, and one of the most learned and influential doctors of his day, had strongly supported the practice of variolation against smallpox. This was a primitive form of inoculation introduced into Europe from the Near East in 1721. Fifty years later Edward Jenner took the first steps towards vaccination.

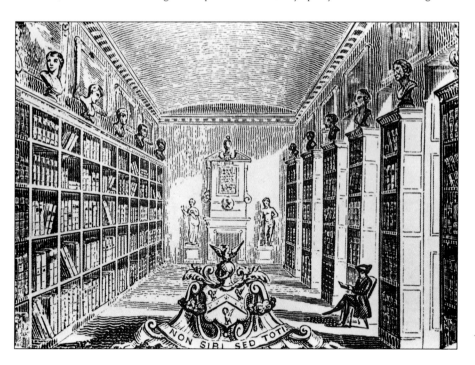

28 Dr Mead's library at No. 49, Great Ormond Street.

29 A painting of the 'Convalescent Ward'. This room was built over the Grand Staircase of No. 48, Great Ormond Street – the house next door to Dr Mead's house into which the hospital expanded in 1858.

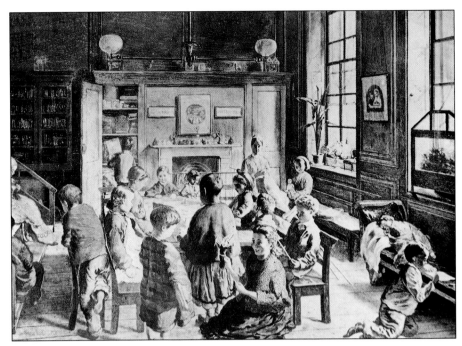

Jenner and vaccination

Edward Jenner was an apprentice to a country surgeon in Gloucestershire when he overheard a dairymaid claim she had no fear of smallpox as she had caught cowpox when milking her herd. Cowpox is a rather rare disease of the cow's teats. It was found only in certain places, and even then only occasionally. Almost at the same time, William Withering discovered digitalis, one of the most important drugs used in heart disease, after learning from an old Shropshire countrywoman that the foxglove was a good cure for dropsy.

Jenner spent many years confirming the truth of the dairymaid's immunity against smallpox. He collected and collated details of similar cases. At last, on 14 May 1796 he made the first crucial vaccination on an 8-year-old boy, James Phipps, with matter taken from a cowpox sore on the hand of Sarah Nelmes, a dairymaid. Seven weeks later, little Phipps was inoculated with the matter of smallpox itself, but he did not take the disease, even when the smallpox inoculation was repeated several months later. This was positive proof. Jenner went on to show that the cowpox vaccine could be passed on from one individual to another without losing its protective powers against smallpox. And, unlike the old system of variolation direct from smallpox itself, there was no danger of developing a serious and sometimes fatal form of the disease.

An unbroken line can be drawn from Jenner through Pasteur to the modern conception of immunology, infection, antibiotics and thence to current and continuing research into the genetic engineering of laboratory-created viruses to use as vaccines against cancer, malaria and AIDS. All vaccines take their name from the Latin for cowpox, *Variolae vaccinae*. Some, like Jenner's cowpox, are the living organisms of a related but minor disease; others are organisms of the original dangerous infection itself, weakened and attenuated in the laboratory to give immunity rather than the

disease. Poliomyelitis, yellow fever, hepatitis (in some forms), typhoid, cholera, diphtheria, whooping cough, and tetanus are some of the diseases now controllable because of the activities of Edward Jenner and James Phipps on that May morning nearly two centuries ago.

Vaccination was quickly put into operation throughout Europe, America and the East, and was soon made compulsory in a number of places. In England, which did not make vaccination compulsory, although the incidence of smallpox was much reduced, the disease was still rightly feared by the public, especially among the poor. This

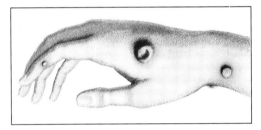

30 The original illustration of cowpox from Edward Jenner's book of 1798.

31 An etching entitled The Cow-Pock *by J. Gillray after himself, 1808. The inscription reads 'The Cow-Pock or the Wonderful Effects of the New Inoculation! ... vide ... the publications of Ye Anti-Vaccine Society'.*

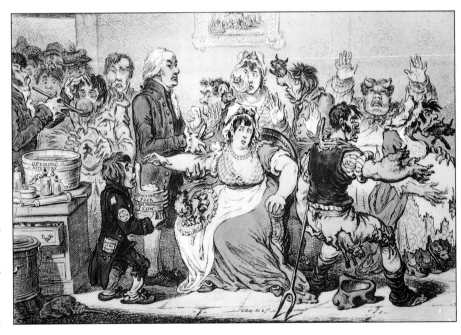

concern found expression when in 1851, six months before Great Ormond Street opened, a Mr Sibley wrote to Lord Shaftesbury seeking an assurance that children with smallpox would not be admitted. The assurance was given. Vaccination was finally made compulsory in England in 1853. By then, however, the great threat to children, as Dr West's first report shows, was scarlet fever.

The threat of epidemic

Another threat, not only to children, was cholera, which first reached Britain in 1831. In 1848, the very year in which Chadwick's Board of Health was established, 54,000 deaths from cholera were recorded. After this epidemic John Snow suggested that the disease was spread by sewage contamination of water supplies. In 1854, during another severe London epidemic of cholera, he gave practical proof of this theory by removing the handle of the Broad Street Pump. Cutting off the infected water supply ended the outbreak of cholera. At that time the germ-borne theory of disease and recognition of disease germs were still unknown.

In 1854, the medical committee at

Great Ormond Street was much concerned with the question of controlling and preventing outbreaks of infection among the children. The outbreak of cholera and summer diarrhoea had put a strain on the out-patients department. The two separate fever wards had, in Dr West's phrase, 'proved themselves' for the in-patients. The practice of seeing new out-patients first to keep them apart while checking for an infectious disease had not always been possible. But thanks to the care and alertness of the medical staff no serious outbreak was to occur. It was decided to follow 'The Examples of the Children's Hospitals in Bremen, Frankfurt, Hamburg, Pest, St Petersburg and Turin', and supply all in-patients with hospital clothing during their stay, and not merely a change of linen. Measles was also a dangerous infection for children. Typhus, typhoid, tuberculosis (in all its forms, not merely that affecting the lungs), diphtheria and whooping cough were some of the other infections with which Great Ormond Street had to grapple, then and later. The story of their conquest is all part of medical history and research, that triumphal march which began with Edward Jenner.

Basic equipment: the beginnings

The story of medicine can also be the story of quite simple things. Most people picture doctors with stethoscopes dangling round their necks or from their pockets, or taking a patient's pulse with a watch. We can hardly conceive a time when stethoscopes and watches, thermometers and hypodermic syringes were not a part of medical equipment. Yet these four everyday items, so essential to medical procedure, came into use quite late in medical history. The young, or even middle-aged, Dr West witnessed their introduction into practice. Although Sir John Floyer had invented the 'Physician's Pulse Watch' in 1707, an instrument which ticked away for exactly one minute, it was not really taken up. Actual watches with second hands mechanically reliable enough to take a pulse were not in general medical use until the nineteenth century.

Hypodermic syringes were invented

by Alexander Wood of Edinburgh and first used in 1853. Thermometers were invented by Galileo around 1593 (he is also credited with first timing a pendulum by his pulse and then his pulse by the pendulum), and sometimes used medically, although only with the greatest difficulty, during succeeding centuries. They only came into practical use in 1867 when Sir Thomas Allbutt of Leeds designed the prototype of the modern clinical thermometer. The stethoscope was the invention of a French physician, René Laennec, in 1819. At first a simple roll of paper, and then a wooden tube about nine inches long, the modern form with a rubber tube leading to each ear belongs to the end of the century.

Great names in medicine

Two of Laennec's most brilliant pupils were the great Dublin physicians Richard James Graves and William Stokes. As well as making other contributions to medical progress, Graves lectured on timing the pulse by the watch and Stokes published an introduction to the stethoscope. In 1838 the young Dr West, fresh from Berlin, spent some months at Meath Hospital in Dublin, where Graves and Stokes were his teachers.

Also in 1838, A. C. E. Barthez and F. Rilliet published the first volume of their *Clinical and Practical Treatise on Diseases of Children* in Paris. The three volumes, completed in 1843, became the greatest French work of the century on the subject. Like that of E. Bouchut after them and C. M. Billard before, both physicians at the Paris children's hospital, it owed much to the Hôpital des Enfants Malades and its facilities for research. The treatises by these four doctors, together with Dr West's *Lectures*, were the most important paediatric textbooks of their time.

When Dr West was studying at Paris in 1837, François Magendie, the founder of modern experimental pharmacy and the science of toxicology, was a dominant influence in the advance of medicine. He and his pupils investigated and isolated the alkaloids, the vital active ingredients of the important vegetable

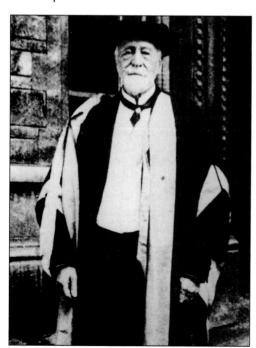

32 Sir Thomas Allbutt of Leeds, who invented the clinical thermometer in 1867.

33 Dr C. M. Billard and Dr E. Bouchut, both working in Paris, made considerable contributions to clinical observation, anatomy and hygiene in the treatment of children.

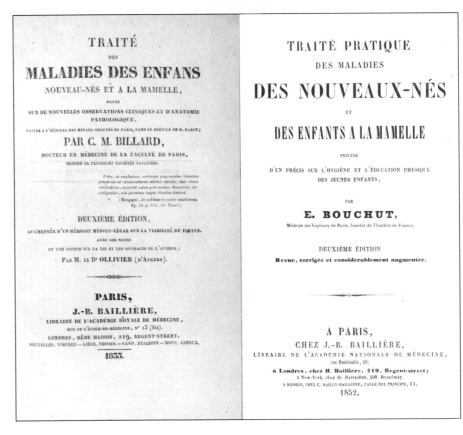

drugs. In Germany, Sertürner had isolated morphine as early as 1806. At Paris, almost within the next decade, Pelletier and Caventour isolated quinine, strychnine and other alkaloids. In 1821 Magendie issued the first formulary for their medical use. This marked the beginning of modern synthetic drugs which have revolutionised medicine and surgery.

As a physiologist, a worker on the functions and structures of organic beings, Magendie was the first of that historical line of laboratory experimenters, of which his greater pupil Claude Bernard, and then Pasteur and Ehrlich were all part. Claude Bernard's work on the physiology of the digestive system, on metabolism and enzymes, and the vasomotor nerves controlling the flow and pressure of the bloodstream, was a fundamental part of that successful exploration of our bodily workings which separate today from the past.

Johannes Müller, Bernard's senior and German counterpart, was perhaps the greatest physiologist of the time. He made important contributions to comparative anatomy, embryology, physiological chemistry (which he practically founded), psychology and pathology. A wonderful teacher, many of his pupils were also famous pioneers in science and medicine. Müller studied and worked at the University of Bonn not long before West studied there, and was professor at Berlin when West received his doctorate

in 1837. His textbook on physiology, a landmark in medicine, first appeared in 1834. A few years later Dr William Baly translated it into English. Baly was West's friend and colleague at St Bartholomew's Hospital. He had also taken his doctorate at Berlin, a year before West; he was a member of Great Ormond Street's first medical committee, and physician to Queen Victoria. On his untimely death in a railway accident, William Jenner, West's colleague at Great Ormond Street, was Baly's immediate successor to the royal post.

Müller was the first to use the microscope in pathology in his great work on tumours and cancerous growths; he gave physicians those diagnostic procedures that are now an integral part of modern clinical procedure: the power to distinguish between benign and malign cells. His book on cancerous growths was based on the concept of the human cell as a fundamental functional unit, a concept developed by him and his pupils Schwann, Henle and Virchow. Müller published the first and only volume of the book in 1838. In 1839 Schwann published

his treatise on cell-growth theory. In 1840 Charles West published the first English translation of Müller's *On the Nature and Structural Characteristics of Cancer*. Five years later Hughes Bennett of Edinburgh and Rudolf Virchow of Berlin first described leukaemia, within a few weeks of each other.

Little serious surgery was done at Great Ormond Street in its early years, except a few amputations of diseased and tuberculous joints, where otherwise the child would have inevitably died. More frequently, surgery was necessary to remove stones from the bladder,

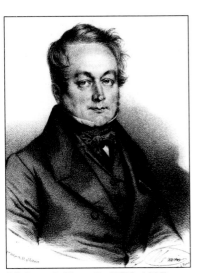

34 François Magendie (1783–1855).

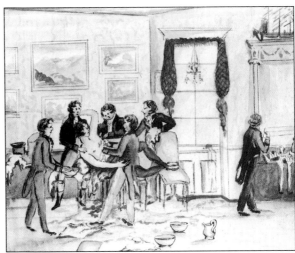

35 Surgery was often carried out in the home!

which the inadequate diet of poor children in those days made quite common. When we think of the great strides made in paediatric surgery at the Hospital for Sick Children, and elsewhere, during the last fifty years, it is instructive to remember that Charles West thought that there were 'no surgical problems in childhood which demanded special skill or study'. But anaesthetics only came into use about two years before Great Ormond Street opened, and antiseptic surgery was not thought of until fifteen years later. Surgery was an agonising and dangerous procedure; even the most skilled and speediest of surgeons were reluctant to inflict this ordeal on a child. Sir Astley Cooper, the greatest surgeon in England, once burst into tears when a little girl, on whom he was to operate, smiled at him as she entered the theatre. Cooper was at the height of his career when West was a young student.

The beginnings of anaesthesia

The first successful operation under general anaesthesia was at Boston, USA, on 16 October 1846, when William Morton used ether in removing a neck tumour. The news crossed the Atlantic and two months later ether was first used in London at the University College Hospital, for the amputation of a thigh. The following January, James Simpson of Edinburgh began to use ether in childbirth. During 1847 the use of ether spread throughout Europe and America.

But ether at that time had certain drawbacks, especially in obstetrics. Simpson sought for a substitute, finding it in chloroform which had been discovered in 1831. In November 1847 Simpson first demonstrated the surgical use of chloroform during an operation on a 5-year-old boy. Although there was some opposition, especially to its use in childbirth, chloroform rapidly became the most widely used and preferred anaesthetic. And when John Snow administered chloroform to Queen Victoria during the birth of Prince Leopold in 1853, the royal example silenced all criticism. In 1848, St Bartholomew's Hospital had wanted Simpson as its new lecturer in midwifery. When he refused to leave Edinburgh for London, Dr West was given the post.

Anaesthesia advanced surgical technique by removing the desperate need for speed and haste – procedures could be considered and deliberate. At Great Ormond Street tracheostomy was the most common emergency operation, slitting open a passage in the windpipe to enable a child being choked with diphtheria to breathe. Instead of the hasty and dangerous deep cuts necessary on a strangling child, a safer and more gradual approach was possible, and a possibly fatal haemorrhage easily avoided. But often the emergency left no time for anaesthesia – the child was already unconscious and choking.

Cleanliness: raising the standards

Although chloroform brought about much surgical progress, the danger of infection, of putrefaction, of festering and suppurating wounds, of hospital gangrene, of blood poisoning – the whole process of what is known as sepsis – was still very great. Nearly half the amputations performed resulted in death. Abdominal operations were not to be thought of. Cleanliness and germs were not understood in this connection. In 1846 Semmelweis had shown that the high mortality from puerperal fever among pregnant patients in a notorious ward at the Vienna Hospital could be reduced from as much as thirty per cent to one per cent by insisting that doctors or anyone examining the women after visiting the post-mortem room should wash their hands. But this obvious and elementary precaution, as it would seem nowadays, was bitterly attacked. It was left to Pasteur to demonstrate the true relation between infection and the existence of germs, and for Joseph Lister of Glasgow to apply Pasteur's findings to solving this last frightful problem of surgery.

Lister turned to the use of carbolic acid as a method of preventing infection from germs in the air, both to wounds in the theatre and when dressing the injury afterwards. On 12 August 1865 an 11-year-old boy, James Greenleas, was admitted to Glasgow Royal Infirmary with a compound fracture of the leg after being run over by a cart. This type of accident, because of the dirt and mud entering the wound, was liable to become badly infected and gangrenous. As an operative procedure carbolic was used to wash the wound and then used in the dressing mixed with a putty of whitening and linseed oil. Six weeks later, James was sent home, still with two whole legs. Lister had proved that antiseptic surgery was feasible and successful, opening the way towards advanced, modern surgery. In 1870 Lister invented his famous carbolic spray, which he used for nearly twenty years. By then surgical technique was aseptic, with all equipment sterilised.

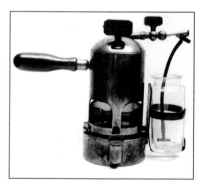

37 A steam-operated Lister carbolic spray.

At Great Ormond Street the first surgical wards date from 1871, but operations must have been performed behind screens, or in a temporary room, as it was only in the new building, opened in 1875, that an operating theatre was fitted out on the top above the chapel. It was in 1877 that a Lister spray is first mentioned in the hospital

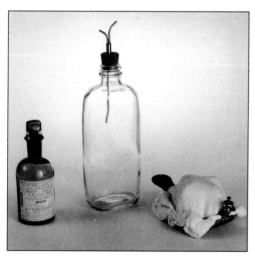

36 An early anaesthetic mask and drip bottle for chloroform used at the Hospital for Sick Children.

records. And in 1878 a first list is given of the operations performed during the year.

Bacteria were first described by the Dutch microscopist, A. van Leeuwenhoek, in 1683. But for centuries their origin was disputed. The theory that maggots and even fair-sized creatures are spontaneously generated from decaying matter was centuries old, as was the theory that contagious diseases and fevers were caused by a strange miasma or vapour rising from the earth. This was held to be responsible for sudden epidemics and outbreaks.

Louis Pasteur

Louis Pasteur, from his work on fermentation (his name is remembered in the pasteurisation of milk), turned to the origin of bacteria. He showed that living micro-organisms existed in the air, causing infection, putrefaction and decay. In 1861 he published his researches. It was the end of the spontaneous generation or miasma theory and the beginning of the germ theory of infection. Pasteur went on to develop the first new vaccines since Jenner and smallpox. He investigated anthrax, and then in 1881 found a method of attenuating the chicken-cholera virus when a culture of the active virus was by oversight forgotten in the laboratory, becoming weakened but still effective as a vaccine against injections of virulent chicken cholera.

Pasteur next sought an inoculation against rabies. Any person then bitten by a mad dog almost certainly faced an agonising death. Pasteur took the saliva from a mad dog and, after passing it first through a rabbit's brain and subsequently into a rabbit's spinal cord, obtained an effective vaccine. On 6 July 1885 a 9-year-old boy, Joseph Meister from Alsace, who had been badly bitten by a mad dog, was the first human to be inoculated against rabies. His life was saved. This put the final seal on Pasteur's fame. Adults and children were sent to Pasteur from all over Europe, including England. The Pasteur Institute was soon founded, and the adult Joseph Meister became its gatekeeper. Sadly, but symbolically, Joseph committed suicide in 1940 when the Nazis occupied Paris

and attempted to force open the crypt where Pasteur was buried.

Although bacteriology was born with Pasteur's work on fermentation, it was Robert Koch, Pasteur's junior by some twenty years, who finally gave bacteriology its predominant position in research with his unrivalled laboratory technique and skill. Koch discovered the anthrax bacillus in 1876; the tubercle bacillus, his most famous achievement, in 1882; and in 1883, the cholera bacillus. He investigated tropical diseases. He evolved the technique of staining bacteria and obtaining pure cultures on glass for microscopical investigation. This, with 'Koch's Postulates', the tests for establishing and locating the presence of the micro-organisms of disease, is still the basic procedure of bacteriology. It was not surprising that at the 1881 International Medical Congress in London Pasteur hailed Koch's work as a great step forward.

Pasteur and Koch, the direct inheritors of that tradition of French and German science which Charles West knew as a student, were in fact the greatest geniuses in the most important of all advances towards modern medicine. Together with Claude Bernard's and

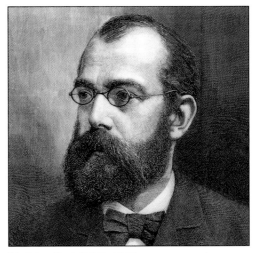

38 Robert Koch (1843–1910) – an engraving by P. Nauman.

Johannes Müller's work on physiology, the development of cell theory by Müller and his pupils, the development of anaesthesia and the control of infection in surgery, their work was the bridge across the divide separating the medicine of today from that of Dr West's boyhood. In 1901, fifty years after the first public meeting to set up a hospital for sick children, Dr George Eastes was appointed the first bacteriologist at Great Ormond Street.

TIME CHART

AD

1590–3 Galileo develops the compound microscope and invents the thermometer.
1683 A. van Leeuwenhoek first sees bacteria under a microscope.
1707 Sir John Floyer designs the 'Physician's Pulse Watch'.
1721 Inoculation against smallpox introduced into Europe.
1785 William Withering: *Account of the Foxglove.*
1796 Edward Jenner vaccinates James Phipps against smallpox.
1800 A. Volta describes effect of electricity on muscles.
1801 K. F. Gauss: *Disquisitiones arithmeticae,* on the theory of numbers. A landmark in mathematics.
1805 F. W. A. Sertürner isolates morphine from opium. The beginning of alkaloid drugs.
1809 F. Magendie begins his investigations into Javanese arrow poison, etc.
1818–20 P. J. Pelletier and J. B. Caventour isolate strychnine, quinine, etc.
1819 R. Laennec invents the stethoscope. Diagnosis by ausculation.
1825 P. Bretonneau performs first successful tracheostomy, and describes and names diphtheria.
1827 Richard Bright publishes his observations on kidney disease.
1831 J. von Liebig discovers chloroform. Cholera first reaches Britain.
1834–40 J. Müller publishes his textbook of physiology, *A Manual of Human Physiology.*
1838 J. Müller: *On the Nature and Structural Characteristics of Cancer.*
1838–43 A. C. E. Barthez and F. Rilliet: *Clinical and Practical Treatise on Diseases of Children.*

1839 T. Schwann's treatise on cell-growth theory.
1845 R. Virchow and H. Bennett first separately describe leukaemia.
1846 W. Morton uses ether as an anaesthetic in Boston. R. Liston follows his example in London. I. P. Semmelweis relates puerperal fever to uncleanliness.
1847 Sir James Simpson uses chloroform as an anaesthetic. Claude Bernard discovers that chemicals are produced in the body.
1848 Board of Health under E. Chadwick in Britain.
1849 John Snow claims cholera is water-borne infection.
1851 Helmholtz invents the ophthalmoscope.
1853 Alexander Wood first uses hypodermic syringe. Vaccination made compulsory in Britain.
1854 John Snow stops a London cholera epidemic by removing the handle of the Broad Street Pump.
1857–61 Louis Pasteur publishes his observations on lactic fermentation and the origin of bacteria; birth of germ theory of infection.
1858 R. Virchow: *Cellular Pathology.*
1859 Charles Darwin: *The Origin of Species.*
1863 Pasteur begins an investigation of silkworm disease.
1865 Lord Lister uses carbolic for antiseptic surgery.
1867 Sir Thomas Allbutt designs prototype of modern clinical thermometer.
1876 Robert Koch discovers the anthrax bacillus.
1880–1 Pasteur develops vaccines against chicken cholera and anthrax.
1882–3 Koch discovers the tubercle bacillus and the cholera bacillus.
1885 Pasteur inoculates Joseph Meister against rabies.

CHAPTER 4

Great Ormond Street to 1914

Great Ormond Street's doctors and nurses

'There was no more touching sight than to see Dr West make his round; the little patients welcomed him as their friend, and the fractious or frightened child could not long resist the magic of his smile or the winning gentleness of his manner.'

These words were written by Catherine J. Wood, Great Ormond Street's revered and influential lady superintendent, or matron, who is remembered in

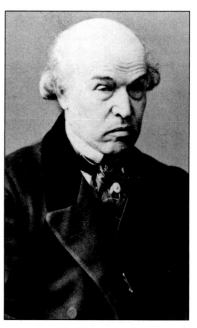

39 Miss Catherine J. Wood, lady superintendent at Great Ormond Street from 1878 to 1888.

its School of Nursing as the founder of modern paediatric nursing and training. Miss Wood had known the hospital since she was a girl living in nearby Doughty Street. She had first been an interested young visitor, then a lady reader to the children in the wards. She helped to divert a child's attention from aches and pains by telling stories, reading from a picture book or writing letters. A little boy undergoing painful treatment promised not to cry if his lady reader would sing to him, which she did. A little girl, her eyes temporarily bandaged, carefully felt a new doll as her lady reader described all the glories of its hair and dress.

Dr West was not alone in his devotion to the children. William Jenner, later Sir William, who shared the medical responsibility for the hospital's first decade, was a masterful personality with stern features and rather terrifying to adults and other doctors. But with the children he was all kindness. One little boy, whose parent was far from handsome, clasped Jenner's hand and looked at him fondly, saying, 'You are so like my daddy!'

Jenner was the first to identify the difference between typhoid and typhus fever. His work at Great Ormond Street produced a valuable treatise on diphtheria. When he became Queen Victoria's personal and trusted physician in 1861, he resigned his Great Ormond Street post but served on its committees for many years. He would sometimes, especially near Christmas, escape from the court at Balmoral or Windsor to spend a happy hour carefully inspecting the toys brought by the Queen and her family for Great Ormond Street, making sure there was nothing among them to harm the patients. Jenner paid tribute to

all that Dr West had done for the Hospital, but Great Ormond Street in many ways owed as much to him.

Dr Thomas Hillier took Jenner's place at Great Ormond Street. He was an early, zealous medical officer of health for St Pancras, and his reports pioneered the prevention of industrial diseases. He retired early, because of ill-health, in 1868. A diet recommended by him for the children included roast beef once a week and green vegetables, if the vegetables were not too expensive; a slice of bread and butter for supper if wanted; and pudding, for convalescents only, three times a week. By the standards of the time, and compared with the boys at Eton and the other great public schools, the children were well fed. Many entered the hospital half-starved and emaciated. The doctors knew that lack of food, let alone of good food, and impure water and foul air were poor children's main enemies.

[Photograph of Dr (later Sir) William Jenner]

40 Dr (later Sir) William Jenner (1815–98).

G. A. Sala, a journalist who had worked with Dickens, described with horror a case of 'starvation' in the girls' ward. 'The face was like a diminutive death's head' and the arm a mere bone, which, the nurse assured him, was 'getting quite plump to what it was a week ago'. Sala, like other visitors, remarked on the expensive toys scattered on cots and tables, 'none of your penny monkeys that run up sticks'. His description of the suffering children, however, coiled up like a ball among the bedclothes, unable to bear the light, or lying stark and rigid, covered with dreadful sores, is a reminder that in the nineteenth century the shocking sights now associated with deprived, backward or famine-stricken countries were seen on London streets.

Nevertheless, the chief impression that most visitors took away was of love and happiness. In 1860 one group of ladies, including a resident of Melbourne, Australia, signed the visitors' book with the comment, 'Much struck with the order and cheerfulness.' In 1861 Mrs Craik, the author of *John Halifax, Gentleman*, wrote, 'Among the fifty sick children in the hospital we heard not a cry or a murmur of fretfulness.' Children were often reluctant to leave the comfort and care of Great Ormond Street to return to the squalor and misery of their homes. One or two children were abandoned by their parents and had to be sent to an orphanage or to Greenwich workhouse.

Dr Frederick Poynton, who retired from the hospital in 1934, commented:

Great Ormond Street seemed to me to be one of the greatest of all charities ... We have to visualise a poor mother with a sick child in one room with perhaps only a basin and ... too many children, or a drunken or out-of-work husband, or one earning but little ... We have to realise that her love for her children was her great happiness in life ... In her trouble she could bring the child to the Hospital.

West's vision of a children's hospital being a powerful social factor for good was as valid in the 1930s as it had been in the 1850s.

After Dr West's retirement in 1875, the principal physicians at Great Ormond Street were William H. Dickinson, Samuel Gee and Walter Butler Cheadle, all men of eminence both there and at their other London hospitals. Dickinson had been at the hospital since 1861. He was known as an authority on kidney disease and on children's diseases. He was highly regarded at St George's

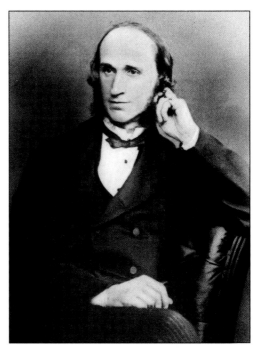

41 Dr Thomas Hillier (1831–68).

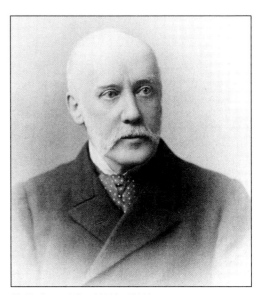

42 Dr Samuel Gee (1839–1911).

Hospital, almost to the point of idolatry. Samuel Gee was the first to identify coeliac disease, also called Gee's disease, a rare but distressing malfunction of the digestive system in infants. In recent years Great Ormond Street has made a special study of this and, with carefully prepared diets and special foods, has done much to overcome the problems. Gee was called the greatest clinician of his time. At St Bartholomew's Hospital he was certainly regarded as a brilliant teacher. At Great Ormond Street, a

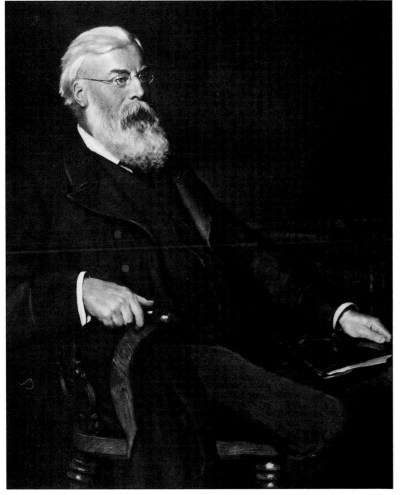

LEFT: *43 Dr William H. Dickinson (1832–1913).*

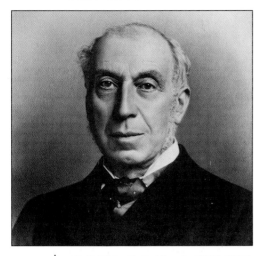

44 *Dr Walter Butler Cheadle (1835–1910).*

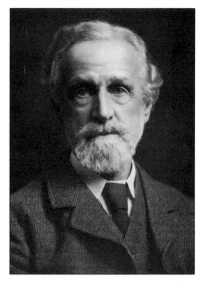

46 *Sir Thomas Smith, surgeon at Great Ormond Street from 1854 to 1910.*

regular Thursday afternoon series of lectures for the medical profession was soon established, its fame and popularity lasting well into the twentieth century.

Childhood diseases defined

In his younger days Cheadle had spent two years with Viscount Milton exploring the Canadian Rockies and the Yukon for a north-west passage by land. They published a book about their travels in 1865. Cheadle, a big man, nearly starved when food ran short in the frozen mountains. To the end of his life he kept the strong leather belt which he had tightened notch by notch. Perhaps it was this experience that led him to discover infantile scurvy. Barlow, his junior at the hospital, continued his work, showing that infantile scurvy was related to adult scurvy and not merely a form of rickets. It became known for a while as Barlow's disease. Cheadle was the first to recognise that rheumatic fever was essentially a disease of childhood. Poynton, his younger colleague and close friend, also did much work in this field; and in 1930, Poynton's own junior colleague, Dr B. Schlesinger, discovered a relationship between throat infections and attacks of acute rheumatic fever. Cheadle was adored by parents and children. It was said that his little patients lay fearlessly in his huge hands, which almost obliterated them, loudly and confidently shouting for a sweet. He was a great champion of women becom-

ing doctors at a time when the old school of thought, to which even West and Jenner belonged, was bitterly opposed to it. Cheadle was one of the first lecturers at the London School of Medicine for Women when it opened in 1874.

Sir Thomas Barlow had first joined Great Ormond Street in 1875 as an assistant physician in the out-patients department. He became one of the most famous and influential doctors of his day; his opinion was often held to be the final judgement in a difficult case. Only a few days before her final illness, Queen Victoria had written that if her doctor, Sir James Reid, needed help, Barlow should be sent for. He told his brother that when he was taken to the Queen's bedside, she greeted him with 'her most charming smile, like that of a child'. Many were the children who smiled at Barlow bending over their cots at Great Ormond Street. When he died in 1945, shortly before his hundredth birthday, he had given them seventy years of un-selfish service as assistant physician, physician, and consulting physician.

These were some of the doctors at Great Ormond Street between 1875 and 1914 – there is no room to list them all. The two leading names in surgery during that time were Sir Thomas Smith and Sir William Arbuthnot Lane. Sir Thomas was trained in the early days of surgery when speed was a necessary skill: he is reported to have extracted a stone from a child's bladder in thirteen seconds. He invented a special gag which allowed cleft-palate operations to be done under

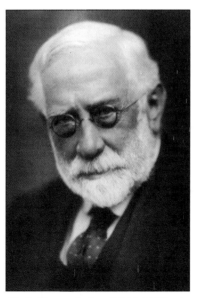

45 *Sir Thomas Barlow (1845–1945), who served the hospital for over seventy years.*

chloroform, thus making it possible to operate on a very young child. Sir William was reputed to be the finest surgeon of his time. He introduced aseptic surgery into the hospital, pioneered the mastoid operation and designed the necessary instruments. This serious operation has been largely avoided in modern times by the timely use of antibiotics. In his later years he concentrated on cleft-palate operations, again devising his own instruments. Great Ormond Street has always been in the forefront of oral surgery. In recent years a team has regularly gone to Sri Lanka to relieve children, and even adults, with hare-lip and other malformations. At Guy's Hospital and Great Ormond Street, Sir William developed a technique of surgical team-work which was well in advance of its time.

An earlier surgeon, Howard Marsh, specialised in orthopaedics. In 1866 he helped Catherine Wood and Joan Perceval, who were then both in charge of wards at Great Ormond Street, to open the Alexandra Hip Hospital in Queen Square, for children with chronic joint complaints. Such children, who needed long-term or permanent treatment, could not be readily accommodated at Great Ormond Street, although some did stay there for many months. This problem troubled others of the hospital's nursing staff. In 1871 the matron, Miss Vizard, and one of the sisters, Miss Graham, left to start the Royal Alexandra Hospital at Rhyl, reputedly the first hospital to advocate open-air treatment for crippled children.

After the cure: convalescence

Great Ormond Street had earlier opened its own convalescent branch at historic Cromwell House near the top of Highgate Hill. Of the fifty-two beds there, twenty were for convalescents, another twenty for chronic surgical cases and twelve for chronic medical cases. On 28 June 1869 the first seventeen boys and girls, aged between 3 and 10, under the charge of two nurses, travelled by private omnibus from Great Ormond Street to Highgate. Many of the children had only known the dreary streets of central London; the

gardens and country around Highgate surprised and delighted them. As they passed the first large open garden, one little girl wanted to know what that beautiful place was. And nearing Cromwell House, another child pointed to the great chestnut trees outside the house and asked, 'What are those big things?'

In the first years of the hospital, children had been sent for convalescence to cottages at Hornsey and Tottenham, then still country; and generous supporters had provided accommodation at Mitcham in Surrey and by the sea in Brighton. For a number of years the hospital reserved a bed or two at the Margate Royal Sea-Bathing Hospital.

Around 1870 a little boy named Willie was admitted with chronic hip disease

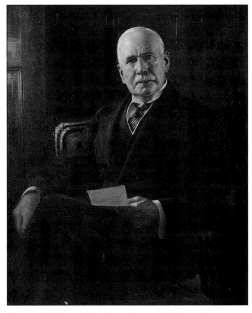

47 Sir William Arbuthnot Lane (1856–1943), surgeon.

LEFT: 48 A ward at Cromwell House.

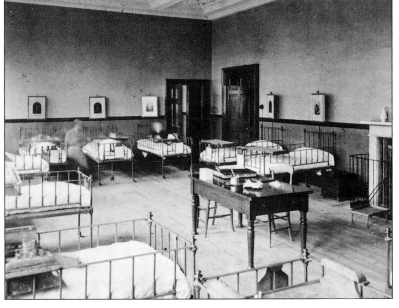

and other complications. He stayed many months at Great Ormond Street and Highgate before being sent to Margate after getting weaker and weaker. On his return to Great Ormond Street, asked how he liked the seaside, Willie replied, 'It was lonely there. You takes a long time to get used to a place, and there ain't no place like this hospital.'

Dr West had persuaded Miss Wood to leave Queen Square and take charge of Cromwell House. After eight years she became matron at Great Ormond Street, where she served another ten years until

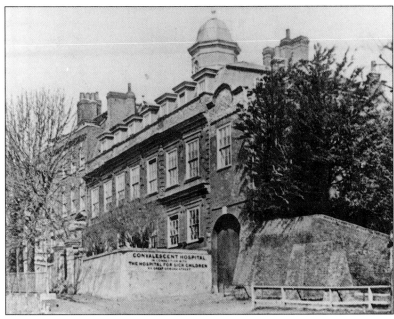

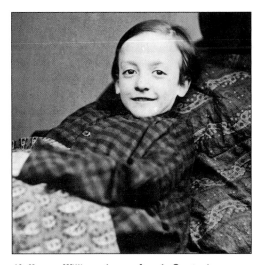

49 Young Willie, who preferred Great Ormond Street to Highgate and Margate!

LEFT: 50 The convalescent branch at Cromwell House, Highgate, London.

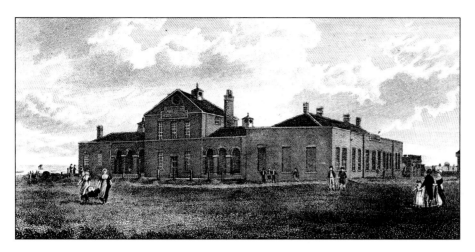

51 The Royal Sea-Bathing Hospital at Margate, where patients from the hospital were sent to recuperate.

1888. She had given over twenty-five years of her life to the children, and, like Miss Vizard and the other devoted women of private means at Great Ormond Street and elsewhere, gave her service free. In the same way, before the passing of the National Health Act in 1946, all the honorary medical staff at Great Ormond Street from West and Jenner onwards not only gave their services without recompense, like the doctors and surgeons at nearly all the great public hospitals, but often drew generously upon their own pockets for the benefit of their own hospital. The fees from their private patients subsidised doctors' hospital work for the poor. In return, the prestige of hospital appointments increased both their reputation and their private practice. At the end of the century the fee for a consultant's visit was three guineas within four miles of Charing Cross. If you lived in the country, calling in a London specialist was something only the well-to-do could afford, as the usual fee was a guinea for every two-thirds of a mile he had to travel. Sir William Jenner, partly because of his prestigious royal appointment, was much in demand for country visits. In his day there were few consultants of recognised status outside London except in the larger, important cities. Jenner left an estate worth £375,000, an enormous sum in those days.

The new breed of nurse

The more humbly paid nurse at Great Ormond Street in its early years received £12 or £20 a year with board.

The work was hard and distressing, the hours long and the living quarters cramped and inadequate. Dr West had set high standards and suitable nurses were hard to find. One of the first to join the hospital was Ann Mooney, an Irish woman older than most. She remained

52 Signatures, including that of Nurse Mooney, in the Nurses' Pay Book (1854).

there for sixteen years, until forced to retire because of increasing arthritis. Several visitors described her over the years in the boys' ward, recalling her treasured collection of photographs pinned over her table. These were of some of the worst cases she had nursed with great skill. The children were fond of their nurses, 'kissing and keeping hold of them with their hands. Nurse Mooney seemed like a dear kind granny among the children.' Dr West's rules for nurses read:

No woman be admitted as a nurse who cannot read readily and write legibly, and who cannot repeat the Lord's Prayer and Ten Commandments ... Mere inability to make children happy will be regarded as of itself a sufficient cause for not retaining a Nurse in the service of the Hospital.

Inspired by Dr West and by Florence Nightingale's example in the Crimea, 'trained and educated gentlewomen' like Miss Wood entered the wards. Among those who sought instruction, or at least spent time helping the children, was Mary Gladstone, daughter of the great prime minister. She told Tennyson about some of her experiences at Great Ormond Street. In 1880 Tennyson published a poem 'In the Children's Hospital', based on Mary Gladstone's story. A sad, sentimental poem about a girl called Emmie, who dies, and Annie, her friend in the next bed, it aroused both support and criticism because of its unsympathetic portrayal of a surgeon. Many years later one lady wrote to Great Ormond Street about her memories of Charles West, whose private patient she had been when a small girl. She described his consulting room in Wimpole Street, where the drawers in his desk were always full of wonderful toys. She and her mother and sisters always knew that 'our kindly old doctor' of Tennyson's poem was a reference to Dr West himself. Certainly Tennyson summed up the whole meaning of Great Ormond Street and its doctors and nurses, Dr West and Sir Thomas Barlow, Ann Mooney and Miss Wood, when he wrote:

I am sure that some of our children would die
But for the voice of love, and the smile, and the comforting eye.

**MATRONS
and
LADY SUPERINTENDENTS
OF THE HOSPITAL**

1852 - 1854	Mrs. WILLEY
1854 - 1861	Mrs. RICE
1862 - 1869	Miss BUBB
1869 - 1871	Miss VIZARD
1871 - 1877	Miss DALRYMPLE HAY
1877 - 1878	Mrs. DICKEN
1878 - 1888	Miss WOOD
1888 - 1890	Miss HICKS
1890 - 1894	Miss CLOSE
1894 - 1897	Miss SMEDLEY
1897 - 1920	Miss PAYNE
1920 - 1935	Miss TISDALE
1935 - 1948	Miss LANE
1948 - 1969	Miss G.M. KIRBY

CHIEF NURSING OFFICERS

1969 - 1975	Miss B.E. CHADNEY
1975 -	Miss B.M. BARCHARD

---

53 Dr West's handwritten notes for nurses.

The new benefactors

Mrs Gatty, the author of many children's stories and the editor of *Aunt Judy's Magazine*, had the then novel idea of endowing a cot at Great Ormond Street with money raised by children who read her magazine. In 1868 an 'Aunt Judy's Magazine Cot' was placed in the girls' ward, the first of its kind not only in Great Ormond Street but in any London hospital. A second cot, for boys, followed in 1876. The £2,000 necessary to endow these cots was raised by the efforts and generosity of children who collected and contributed their pennies. This was a remarkable foreshadowing of the great part played by children in the overwhelming success of Great Ormond Street's recent Wishing Well Appeal.

But long before that appeal, children once again demonstrated their personal affection and concern for Great Ormond Street by collecting £5,910 for the

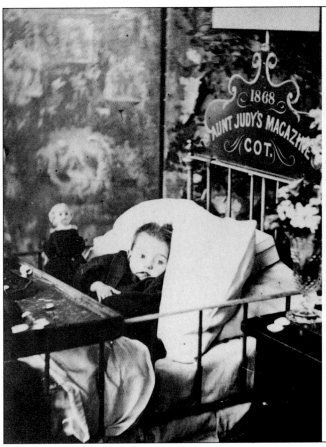

CHRISTMAS IN A HOSPITAL.

AMONG several letters of inquiry and remark upon the subject of the "Aunt Judy Cot" in 49, Great Ormond Street, comes one which induces us to throw our various items of information together under the above heading.

It is not an inviting title, however, we must admit. Even the kindest of happy and *well* children—those most ready to give of their pocket-money to help the sad sick ones—would like to forget, for Christmas time at any rate, that there are those others going through pain and suffering.

It is a natural feeling, and grown-up people share it. Nor does God wish us to shut our eyes to the happiness He permits us to enjoy for a time, by a perpetual dwelling upon burdens, which, though our neighbours' lot to-day, may be ours to-morrow. But it is quite another thing to inquire how far the sick and sad little-ones may be comforted and have their trials alleviated, and into this no one need be afraid to look. For surely even the happiest of the *well* children will be made additionally happy by finding that the ill ones can have a share in happiness and enjoyment.

"Daisy" asks if the sick children are allowed "tea with bread and butter," as she has, and whether they have *cake and oranges at Christmas.* Now we were not able ourselves to answer "Daisy's" question in full, so we sent her letter to Mr. Whitford, the secretary, and from him learn the following particulars :—

All children entering the hospital are attended by a medical man, who, after considering their case, appoints a certain *diet* for them ; *i.e.*, he orders the sort of food which will do them most good. Of these

54 *Aunt Judy's Magazine Cot, endowed in 1868, was the first of its kind.*

55 *Architect's drawing of the South Wing, added in 1893, which still stands in Great Ormond Street.*

Children's Jubilee Tribute in honour of Queen Victoria's golden jubilee. With the Queen's permission this was devoted to the building of a South Wing to the hospital, which had been planned for the 1875 building but abandoned because of insufficient funds. The old original hospital houses at 49 and 48, Great Ormond Street, were demolished, and on 4 June 1893 the Prince and Princess of Wales opened the new wing. The ceremony was marked by the presentation to the Princess of 131 purses donated towards the hospital. Each donor had selected a child to make the presentation, and these included patients from the hospital, some having to be carried in their nurses' arms. The Princess of Wales brought a toy for every

child in the hospital, and went through all the wards handing them out.

Two years later the plans for the hospital, as originally conceived by Barry twenty-five years before, were at last completed. New wards for infectious

56 *One of the silk purses presented to HRH Princess Alexandra, which is now in the Peter Pan Gallery – the museum of the hospital – together with a sailor suit worn by one of the children making a donation.*

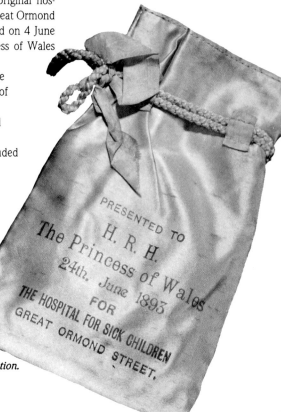

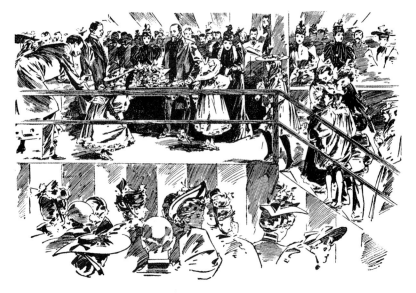

57 An engraving from the Daily Graphic *showing children presenting purses to HRH Princess Alexandra on 24 June 1893. The boy in the sailor suit is seen ascending the steps on the right.*

diseases, including diphtheria and whooping cough, were added to the North Block, which had been left unfinished in 1877. The entire cost of this work and of equipping the new wards was donated by two sisters, the Misses Cohen, as a memorial to their niece, the Countess of Rosebery.

With the development of cheap public transport, children from the suburbs were easily brought to Great Ormond Street. Every poor mother was anxious to bring her sick child there. In 1904 the hospital still stressed in its regulations that 'it is intended for the *Poor* only'. That meant, in effect, children whose parents did not earn more than £2 a week. At that time the average agricultural worker's wage was considerably

less than £1 a week, so nearly every poor child could be accepted without question. In any case, it was only after a first visit that questions were asked about the parents' income. Even then, as the old and long-retired Dr West pointed out in 1896, the rule was far from rigidly kept. All this threw a great strain on the out-patients department in the basement of the 1875 building. Originally designed for a maximum daily attendance of 150 cases, by 1903 the daily total frequently reached 600. In the same year, 2,403 children were admitted as in-patients and 945 operations were performed. Twenty-five years before, in 1878, there had been only 1,058 in-patients and only 82 operations.

It was evident that Great Ormond

Street was now not only taking children from the whole of London and the home counties, but, as the records confirm, from all over England. The out-patients department, once so spacious and ample for all needs, became more and more crowded. The conditions alarmed the medical staff, who feared that the crammed basement would bring infection to the wards above. The council of the King Edward's Hospital Fund repeatedly urged the building of a new department separated from the main building, but the hospital could not afford it. In 1902 the Annual Report wondered if 'in these days of millionaires and magnificent benefactions . . . some of these may cast a compassionate eye'. A response was not long in coming.

William Waldorf Astor gave £50,000 for a new out-patients building as a memorial to his 8-year-old daughter Gwendoline Enid, who had recently died from tuberculosis. He also contributed towards the purchase of the site next to

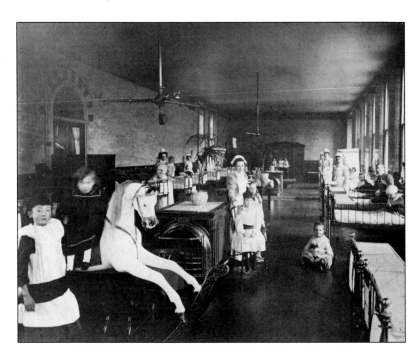

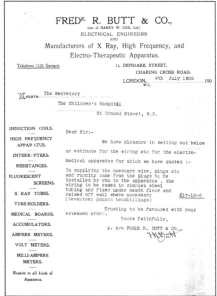

58 Electricity was installed in the operating theatre in 1898. Over the next few years it was gradually fitted to the rest of the hospital. Electrical apparatus for treatment was also first used about this time, as this estimate for equipment, dated 9 July 1909, shows.

59 A ward in the hospital, c. 1890, before the gas lighting had been replaced by electricity.

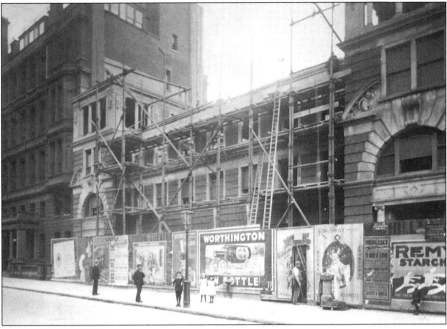

60 The Astor Out-patients Department under construction (1907).

Other children's hospitals

The contributions made by other children's hospitals and their doctors should not be forgotten, even if there is only room to mention a few names. Dr Louis Borchardt, exiled from Berlin, settled in Manchester and worked at its General Dispensary for Children in 1854. The first six beds for in-patients were probably in use by 1855; twenty-five beds became available at new premises in Bridge Street during 1860. The greatly enlarged Manchester Children's Hospital was built at Pendlebury in 1870. The Manchester children benefited from Dr Borchardt for twenty-five years. Dr Henry Ashby, who came to Pendlebury in 1879, stayed for nearly thirty years. For many years he lectured on paediatrics at the University of Manchester, effectively promoting infant welfare and a pure milk supply. With George Wright, surgeon to the Manchester Royal Infirmary, he collaborated on a treatise on the medical and surgical diseases of children, the first such joint effort. Another German specialist in children's diseases, Abraham Jacobi, was imprisoned in Germany for political reasons,

the hospital. The Astor Building was opened in 1908. The main waiting hall had room for 500 children with their mothers. In a few years, with well over 100,000 appointments every year, it was one of the largest and busiest departments in the world. Over 3,000 patients were also admitted annually and nearly 2,000 operations performed.

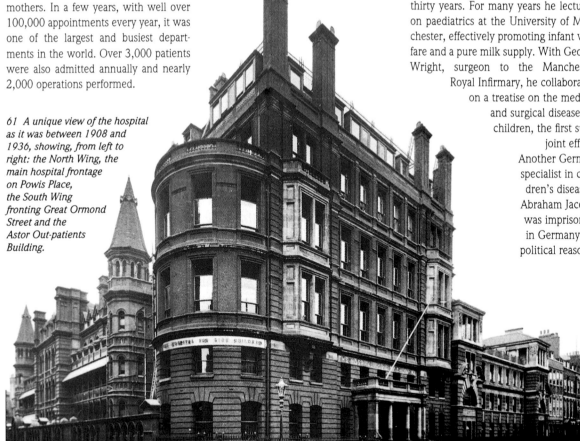

61 A unique view of the hospital as it was between 1908 and 1936, showing, from left to right: the North Wing, the main hospital frontage on Powis Place, the South Wing fronting Great Ormond Street and the Astor Out-patients Building.

62 Hôpital des Enfants Malades, established in Paris in 1802 – the first children's hospital in Europe.

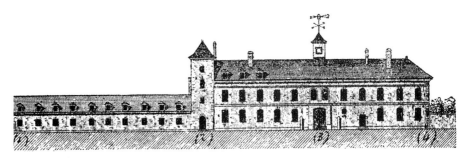

eventually escaping to America in 1853. He was America's leading authority on paediatrics for more than fifty years. He thought Dr West's lectures on children's diseases easily the best work of their time. William Northrup and Samuel Adams were two other doctors who contributed much to the advance of children's hospitals in the USA, becoming professors of paediatrics at New York and Washington.

Dr Alfred Stephens of Liverpool visited Great Ormond Street to study its methods and organisation. He made use of its diet sheets when he opened his children's hospital with eight beds at Hope Street, Liverpool, in 1857. The foundation stone for the Royal Liverpool Children's Hospital was laid in Myrtle Street on 3 February 1869. Thirty years later, two leading orthopaedic surgeons, Sir Robert Jones and Charles Macalister, opened the Royal Liverpool Country Hospital for Children, where chronic disabled children could receive the lengthy and extensive treatment they needed. Other children's hospitals had opened elsewhere in London apart from Great Ormond Street, and also in Leeds, Sheffield, Birmingham, Edinburgh, Glasgow, Newcastle and many other places.

In Germany, Carl Henning founded his Dresden Children's Hospital in 1863. Carl Gerhardt, the greatest German paediatrician of his day, was professor at Jena in 1861 and at Berlin from 1863. His great compendium of children's diseases, which he edited in sixteen volumes between 1877 and 1896, ranks with the French work by Rilliet and Barthez, mentioned in the previous chapter, as the authoritative source for historical data on children's diseases. Gerhardt made a valuable contribution to the study of laryngology. Johann Steffen was physician at the children's hospital in Stettin from 1853 to 1900. Like Dr Mauthner of Vienna, who had advised Dr West on the setting up of Great Ormond Street, Steffen was one of a number of German doctors who established their own children's hospitals.

Eduard Heinrich Henoch was director of the paediatric clinic at the Charité Hospital, Berlin. He translated Dr West's *Lectures* in 1872, wrote much on children's diseases himself and, like Dr West, was noted for his classic and exquisite style. He gave his name to Henoch's purpura, a serious children's gastro-intestinal disorder marked by livid purple spots on the stomach.

Karl Rauchfuss and Nil Filatov in Russia were directors of the children's hospitals at St Petersburg and Moscow during the last quarter of the century. Both contributed greatly to the problem of infectious diseases in children and their control in hospital. Here paediatrics set an instructive example for general medicine. In Paris in 1904, Victor-Henri Hutinel of the Hôpital des Enfants Malades was the first to design an isolation cubicle of transparent glass screens with doors and an aseptic procedure for entry and exit. There was soon scarcely a hospital in the world that did not make use of them.

Children's hospitals were similarly responsible for abandoning the old, strict, regimented approach to patients in hospital. That the relationship everywhere between patients and their doctors and nurses is now more relaxed, sympathetic and understanding, is something we owe to Dr West and his fellow-paediatricians.

TIME CHART

AD

1754 Dorothea Erxleven first woman to receive a medical degree, in Germany.
1849 Elizabeth Blackwell and Sarah Dolly first women medical graduates in USA.
1850 Women's Medical College founded in Philadelphia.
1852 Dr Charles West and Sir William Jenner first physicians at Great Ormond Street. George Pollock first surgeon at Great Ormond Street, resigns 1853.
1853 Athol Johnson surgeon at Great Ormond Street.
1853 Dr Abraham Jacobi arrives in America.
1854 Dr Louis Borchardt settles in Manchester.
1855 Dr C. M. Babbington and Dr J. M. Reynolds physicians at Great Ormond Street.
1856 Samuel Cartwright junior, a friend of Charles Dickens, dental surgeon at Great Ormond Street.
1857 Dr T. Hillier physician at Great Ormond Street.
1859 Timothy Holmes surgeon at Great Ormond Street.
1861 Jenner appointed Queen Victoria's personal physician. Sir Thomas Smith surgeon at Great Ormond Street. Dr W. H. Dickinson physician at Great Ormond Street.
1864 Charles Dickens begins publication of *Our Mutual Friend*, containing tribute to Great Ormond Street.

1865 Elizabeth Garrett Anderson first woman in Britain granted licence to practise medicine.
1868 *Aunt Judy's Magazine* Cot for Girls.
1869 Cromwell House, Highgate, opened as convalescent branch.
1870–8 Miss Catherine Wood lady superintendent at Cromwell House.
1874 London School of Medicine for Women opened.
1875 Sir Thomas Barlow physician at Great Ormond Street.
1876 *Aunt Judy's Magazine* Cot for Boys.
1878–88 Miss Wood lady superintendent at Great Ormond Street.
1880 Tennyson publishes poem 'In the Children's Hospital'.
1884 Sir William Arbuthnot Lane surgeon at Great Ormond Street.
1893 South Wing opened by Prince and Princess of Wales.
1894 First glass isolation cubicles designed in Paris.
1899 Sir Frederic Still physician at Great Ormond Street.
1906 Dr F. E. Batten physician at Great Ormond Street.
1908 Astor Out-patients Building opened.

CHAPTER 5

The Pioneers of Modern Medicine and the Beginnings of Team Research

The fight against diphtheria

One hundred years ago, on Christmas Day 1891, Emil von Behring injected a child in a Berlin hospital with an anti-diphtheria serum. The fight had begun against one of the most dangerous childhood diseases, a disease that could also imperil adults. A great step forward in medicine, it showed that bacteriology could find a cure for an established disease which had previously baffled medicine and science. The anti-toxin serum discovered by von Behring and Kitasato, his fellow researcher from Japan, worked by uniting with the diphtheria toxin already in the blood and making it harmless. It was the first of several such serums which became the only cures then known for other infections, including tetanus and gangrene. They were also used against diseases such as pneumonia and meningitis but with only moderate success. Von Behring's anti-toxins, later modified into even safer forms called toxoids, were to make new and successful immunisation programmes possible; diphtheria is now virtually eliminated in the West. Pupils of both Pasteur and Koch had worked on the diphtheria toxin and serum, thus forging another link in the advancing chain of medical progress.

Diphtheria was a disease known to the ancients. Hippocrates possibly described it, and the Romans certainly knew it as the Egyptian or Syrian ulcer of the throat. The Hebrew Talmud, from around AD 400, called it *askara*, 'a much dreaded epidemic disease which usually attacks children, is located in the throat, and kills the patient by a painful death from suffocation'. At its first report in a Hebrew community the neighbourhood was warned by urgently sounding the *shofar* or trumpet; this was not unlike the large bell still preserved in an English children's hospital which in the old days rang out to warn the nearest surgeon that a child was choking with diphtheria and a tracheostomy was imperative.

The first such successful operation was performed by a French surgeon, Pierre Bretonneau, on 1 July 1825 on a girl named Elizabeth de Puységur, after five previous failures. It was Bretonneau who named the disease diphtheria, making the first true clinical distinction between it and scarlet fever, with which it was often confused.

Epidemics of diphtheria had often broken out. The belief that it was caused by bad smells was not easily given up, even after the acceptance of Pasteur's germ theory. At Great Ormond Street there were several outbreaks. In 1880 it was blamed on the demolition of some neighbouring houses. Windows were kept closed and eventually a whole ward shut down for some time. Another outbreak in 1889 led to extensive examination of the drains. But in 1884 Edwin Klebs and Friedrich Loeffler had discovered the diphtheria bacillus and obtained a pure culture; and in 1888, at the Pasteur Institute, Roux and Yersin began filtering and attenuating it, following the earlier precedent of chicken cholera. In 1889, while Great Ormond Street was checking its drains to prevent diphtheria, two of Koch's assistants, von Behring and Kitasato, began their decisive experiments with diphtheria anti-toxin. By 1892 the anti-diphtheria serum was commercially available and it was generally used for treatment from about 1895.

Patients' statistics at Great Ormond Street demonstrate what a great blessing von Behring had provided. In 1894 there were eighty-one cases of diphtheria, forty-four of whom died. In 1896, a year after the new treatment began to be widely used, seventy-eight cases of diphtheria were admitted, but only ten died. By 1904 there were only thirty-six cases with only three deaths.

Paul Ehrlich, another dominant figure in bacteriology and medical progress, worked with von Behring, determining the necessary quantities, refinement and effect of the diphtheria anti-toxin. His investigation became a classic of immunology. An explanation of how the body's immunological defences worked had been put forward by Elie Metchnikoff, a Russian pathologist who joined the Pasteur Institute as a sub-director in 1887. He described how certain white cells in the blood, the phagocytes, could

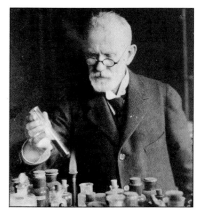

63 Paul Ehrlich (1854–1915) in his laboratory.

engulf and absorb invading particles and bacteria. Metchnikoff and Ehrlich were jointly awarded the Nobel Prize in 1908 for their 'work on immunity'.

Ehrlich knew, however, that the serums and vaccines available were not always the best answer to diseases and infections, and too many of those still had no certain cure. His early interest in chemistry, his experience in using synthetic aniline dyes to stain cells for microscopic examination and investigation, and his work on the diphtheria antitoxin and the molecular structure of protoplasm made him believe he could find a synthetic chemical whose molecules would act on specific microorganisms of disease, without harming the host body. Chemotherapy, which Ehrlich was to prove possible, is one of the most important tools of modern medicine. He first used the term 'chemotherapy' in 1905, the year in which he made important pioneer discoveries on cancer cells, and in which the bacillus of whooping cough was isolated by Bordet and Gengou. It was also the year in which Schaudinn discovered the microparasite of syphilis, the next problem Ehrlich tackled.

A remedy for syphilis

From the first, Great Ormond Street had children with congenital syphilis which had been passed on to them at birth by an infected mother. More were treated as out-patients: 118 in 1876, of whom nearly 80 were not yet 2 years old. Their position must have been

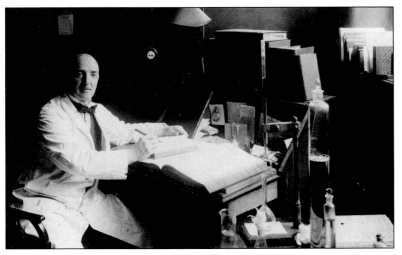

similar to children suffering from AIDS today. There was not much that could be done for them – of seven children admitted in 1900 with congenital syphilis, five died. People regarded them with the same prejudice born of ignorance and fear of infection that we see today. And some parents were certainly worried about the presence of syphilitic children in the Great Ormond Street wards.

Ehrlich first experimented with the aniline dye, trypan red; he then turned his attention to an arsenical drug, Atoxyl, of which by 1907 he had made and tested over 600 compounds. The 606th preparation was at first wrongly reported to be ineffective against the syphilis parasite. But when re-tested in 1910 by Ehrlich's new Japanese assistant, S. Hata, it was found to be very active indeed.

Team research

Medical and scientific advance was no longer confined to the brilliant individual researcher, but was more and more the province of a group of researchers working as a team. Genius, in the person of another Pasteur, Koch or Ehrlich, would still lead and point the way, but team research was becoming the valid method of seeking out the hidden and more complicated secrets of nature.

'606' or Salvarsan, as the new drug was called, became, before penicillin, the first effective remedy for syphilis. It replaced mercury (which was originally used by Paracelsus in the sixteenth century) with its dangerous, unpleasant

side-effects. As Dr Duthie of the Lister Institute said in 1946, Salvarsan had given 'new health and freedom from fear to hundreds of thousands of victims of one of the greatest scourges which has ever afflicted humanity'. Salvarsan also cured yaws, a contagious tropical disease, mostly affecting children, especially poor children, with disfiguring swellings and sores on their faces, toes and genitals.

That the female mosquito carried the malaria parasite was demonstrated by Ronald Ross in India in 1898. A few years later, Walter Reed in Cuba proved the mosquito also carried yellow fever. Control of these two widely spread and deadly tropical fevers was now possible. Until 1864 a milder form of malaria, known as ague, was common on the Kent and Essex marshes near London. In Great Ormond Street's early years some children were admitted with this fever, but reclaiming of land on the river banks brought about the disappearance of malaria in London. Another fever was controlled when vaccination against typhoid was introduced, first in France in 1888, and then in a more practical form by Almroth Wright to the British Army in India and South Africa around 1900.

The discovery of X-rays and radium

Before Wilhelm Röntgen discovered X-rays in 1895, doctors and surgeons were in many ways like half-blind men groping in the dark. Injured bones and internal organs, abnormalities and deficiencies could now actually be seen for the first time. Some years were to pass and the apparatus greatly improved before all the possibilities of X-rays could be used. At Great Ormond Street the head pharmacist, J. W. Peck, following the example of many early experimenters, took sample X-ray photographs of his hand. In 1902, the same year as the Middlesex Hospital first opened its separate X-ray department, the board decided 'the establishment of a Röntgen Ray department has become a necessity', and by 1903 Dr Morton Smart became Great Ormond Street's first radiographer.

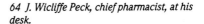

64 J. Wicliffe Peck, chief pharmacist, at his desk.

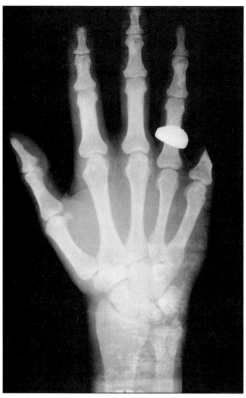

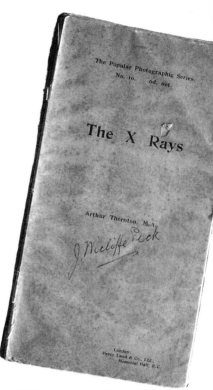

Apart from their great help in diagnosis, X-rays were to prove useful in many ways. Radiology was one development. When Sir Laurence Bragg and his father discovered the law of X-ray diffraction around 1914, it was possible to determine the exact order and array of atoms in a crystalline structure. This helped in the research for new synthetic drugs. Insulin was improved by this method, to the great relief of all diabetics.

The first viruses, particles so small that they passed through filters which could separate bacteria, were found in 1892 and 1898 to be the cause of disease in tobacco plants and of foot-and-mouth disease in cattle. They are now known to be the cause of influenza, smallpox, measles and many other infections. But until the appearance of the electron-microscope, viruses could not be properly seen or studied.

In 1898, Marie and Pierre Curie discovered radium, which became an important element in radiotherapy and the treatment of cancer. But a number of the early workers in radium and X-rays were insufflciently shielded and fell victims to the cancer they were helping to relieve. Radiation influenced and created much of modern physics. When the Nobel Prizes were first awarded, in 1901, Röntgen won the prize for

67 The complete radiographer's handbook for 1896! Written by Arthur Thornton, science master at Bradford Grammar School, and published in the Popular Photographic Series by Percy Lund & Co., just one year after Röntgen published his paper 'On a new kind of Rays'.

physics; the prize for medicine went to von Behring. The Curies shared the physics prize in 1903.

65 Radiography began to spread as a 'hobby' even to the extent of a published handbook. J. Wicliffe Peck, chief pharmacist to the hospital 1896–1936, took what is probably the first radiograph taken at Great Ormond Street, of his own hand.

BELOW: *66 Taking a chest X-ray in 1921. The radiologist is Dr Shires.*

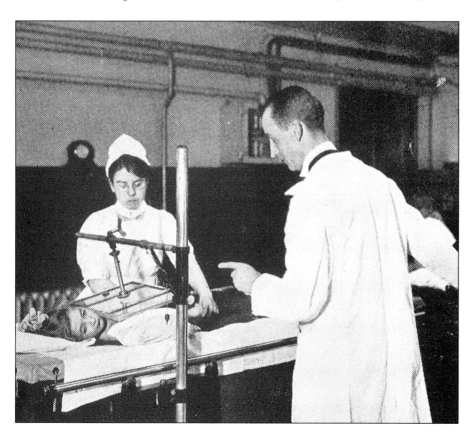

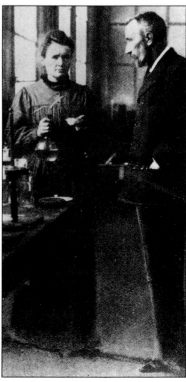

68 Drs Marie and Pierre Curie in their laboratory.

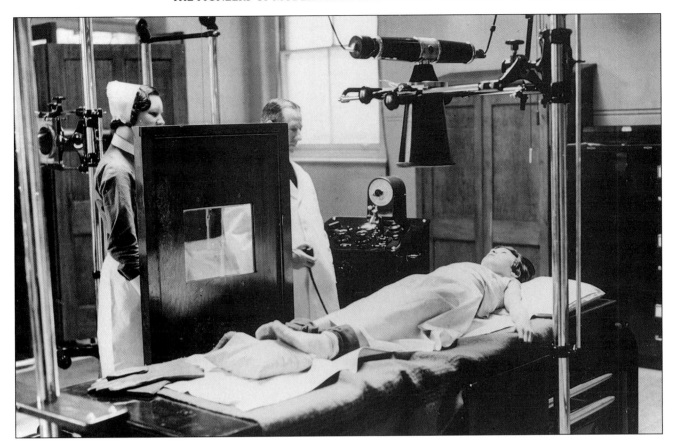

Great strides in surgery

Surgery had made great strides forward, Theodor Billroth in Vienna extending its field more than anyone. He was the first to remove the larynx and in 1881 he successfully cut out part of the upper stomach for cancer. Victor Horsley at the National Hospital, London, pioneered the first removal of a tumour from the brain, developing the art of neurosurgery. There has always been a strong link between the staff of the National Hospital and neighbouring Great Ormond Street, which did not have its specialist neurosurgeon until Wyllie McKissock was appointed in 1939. Cocaine, novocain, barbitone and various barbiturates were introduced as pain-killers and sedatives in the twenty years from 1885, and as a consequence anaesthetics were developed for administration by injection. Dressler produced synthetic aspirin in 1899.

The sphygmomanometer for measuring blood pressure was invented in 1896, and the electrocardiograph, which recorded the heart's tiny electrical impulses, in 1903. Blood transfusion, although already in use, was only made safe when Karl Landsteiner discovered blood-groups in 1901. These three things were to be important in the later development of intensive care which kept alive the premature baby and the seriously ill or injured child or adult.

Vitamins, so vital a part of nutrition and the maintenance of health, especially in the young, became known about 1912. Hormones, those internal secretions carried in the blood which excite a

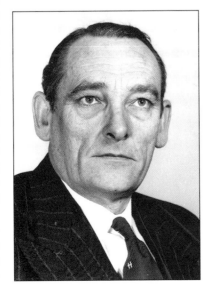

70 Sir Wyllie McKissock, first neurosurgeon to the hospital (born 1906).

specific organ and regulate much of the body's chemistry, were first identified in 1905. It was the start of the modern study of endocrinology and the realisation of the important role played by enzymes and their control by the genetic code. It was a shift in the concept of medicine and disease, and something on which much work is being done at Great Ormond Street as it can answer many hitherto insoluble problems affecting babies and children.

A revolution in psychology

A revolution in psychology also occurred at the turn of the century, in 1900, two years after Dr West's death. That year Sigmund Freud published his *Interpretation of Dreams*, which analysed dreams as revealing the importance of forgotten and unconscious emotions and desires, most of which originated in childhood. This book founded the school of psychoanalysis.

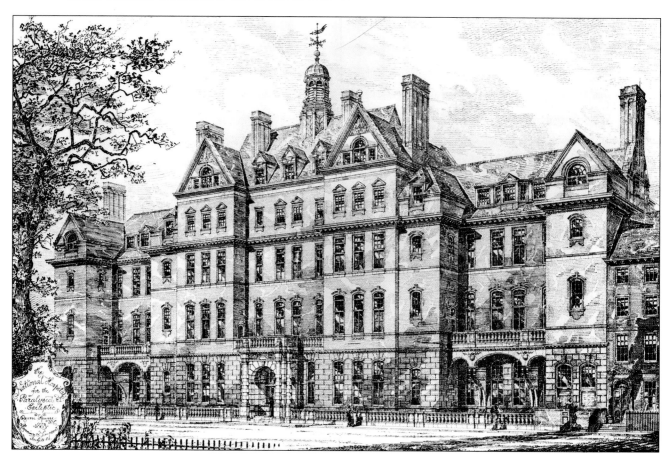

71 *The National Hospital for the Paralysed and Epileptic, now the National Hospital for Neurology and Neurosurgery, stands in Queen Square adjacent to the Hospital for Sick Children.*

Dr West was greatly interested in what he called the nervous disorders of childhood. He emphasised the difference between the adult's mind and the child's. Children may lack the normal adult's power of reason and logic, but they have especially vivid imaginations and emotions. They can love or hate intensely without cause or reason, and are liable to suffer extreme dread or terror. Dr West said all this showed especially in their nightmares and vivid dreams; with his natural sympathy for children he was far in advance of the psychiatric medicine of his time. In some ways he anticipated Freud, although it is doubtful that Dr West would have agreed with all his theories. What would have pleased West was that Freud's daughter, Anna, who came to London with her father in 1938, was a pioneer of child psychoanalysis, and that Great Ormond Street now has its own extensive and influential Department of Psychological Medicine.

TIME CHART

AD

1825 Pierre Bretonneau performs first successful tracheostomy and names 'diphtheria', distinguishing it from scarlet fever.
1870–81 T. Billroth performs first surgical extirpations of larynx, gullet and upper stomach for cancer.
1872–87 J. M. Charcot lectures on nervous diseases at Paris. Sigmund Freud attends in 1885 and is deeply influenced.
1883 Elie Metchnikoff introduces phagocytic theory of immunity.
1884 E. Klebs and F. Loeffler discover diphtheria bacillus.
1885–1905 Cocaine, novocain, barbitone and barbiturates used as pain-killers and sedatives.
1887 Elie Metchnikoff joins Pasteur Institute. Paul Ehrlich formulates side-chain theory of toxins.
1891 Emil von Behring first uses anti-diphtheria serum. Victor Horsley removes a tumour from the brain.
1895 Wilhelm Röntgen discovers X-rays.
1896 Sphygmomanometer invented.
1898 Marie and Pierre Curie discover radium. First viruses investigated. Sir Ronald Ross shows female mosquito carries malaria parasite.

1899 Dreisler processes synthetic aspirin.
1900 Walter Reed demonstrates that yellow fever is carried by mosquito.
c. 1900 Sir Almroth Wright inoculates British Army against typhoid.
1901 First Nobel Prizes for medicine and physics won by Behring and Röntgen.
1903 W. Einthoven invents electrocardiograph. The Curies share Nobel Prize for Physics.
1904 I. P. Pavlov awarded Nobel Prize for work on physiology of digestion, Pavlov's conditioned reflexes.
1905 Bordet and Gengou isolate whooping cough bacillus. Schaudinn discovers micro-parasite of syphilis.
c. 1905 Hormones first named and studied.
1908 Metchnikoff and Ehrlich share Nobel Prize for work on immunity.
1910 Ehrlich discovers Salvarsan '606', a remedy for syphilis.
c. 1912 Vitamins become known.
1914 Sir William Bragg and his son, Sir Laurence, discover law of X-ray diffraction.

CHAPTER 6

The Next Thirty Years

The hospital in wartime

With the outbreak of the First World War in August 1914, most of the other London hospitals soon cut down on, or even completely abandoned, their treatment of children. Room had to be made for the large numbers of wounded returning from the Front. This threw a great strain on Great Ormond Street's staff and resources, already under pressure. The younger doctors had all volunteered for army service. To replace some of them, for the first time in the hospital's history, 'Medical Women' were appointed to resident medical and surgical posts.

Then in 1914, Dr George Pirie arrived from Canada. His wife had died and he decided to come to England and join the Hospital for Sick Children as resident medical officer. He had already done much work at children's hospitals in New York. With his experience and what a colleague described as 'stupendous power of working', he became the mainstay of the hospital during the war and the difficult years immediately afterwards. After six years he returned to Canada to become physician to the Toronto Children's Hospital and its associate professor of paediatrics. North America and Great Ormond Street never forgot these old ties.

It was during the war that parents first made a contribution, according to their means, towards the cost of keeping their children in the hospital. It was no longer strictly a hospital for sick children of the poor. But many of the children admitted still came from penniless families, so its original charitable purpose was not lost, as some of its older staff had feared. The wealthier classes, young and old, were still treated, and even operated on, at home. But for some time surgeons and doctors had been insisting that only properly equipped and maintained premises could offer effective treatment, and had started their own private nursing homes and hospitals. For years, Great Ormond Street had supplied trained children's nurses to private patients. During 1904, for example, the private nursing staff had earned the hospital over £2,300 in fees. And wealthy parents, whose children had been nursed through serious illnesses, usually became generous patrons of the hospital. But it was

72 A photograph taken in one of the wards, probably between 1910 and 1915.

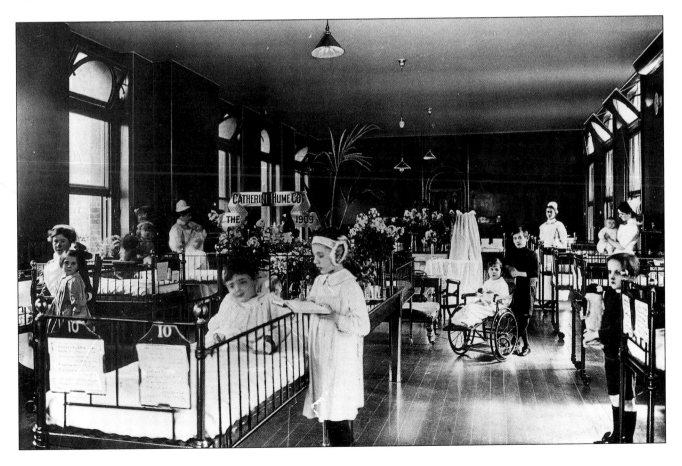

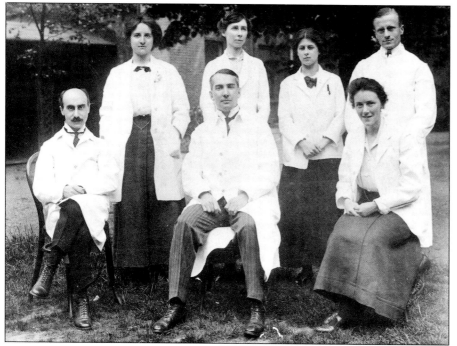

not until 1938 that private beds became available at Great Ormond Street.

Immediately after the First World War, during 1918–19, a terrible influenza epidemic ravaged the world. It caused nearly 20 million deaths, more than twice the total of 8½ million killed in the armed forces of all the combatants during four years of war. Many children caught influenza, but during its most severe wave in 1919 it attacked mostly youths and young adults, who often died within one or two days. Influenza swept through Great Ormond Street, striking down the staff. The children mostly escaped infection, thanks to the self-sacrifice of devoted nurses. Three sisters died of influenza within a fortnight, and as Dr Poynton remembered, 'For the first time I saw the nursing staff on the point of panic, but they rallied and the wave passed away.'

A country hospital

The war and conscription confirmed what the Boer War had revealed fifteen years before – a large part of the adult population suffered ill-health and

had poor physique, the result of a bad or inadequate diet, untreated bodily ailments and unhealthy living conditions, all dating from childhood. In 1890 the London School Board had appointed a medical officer for children. By 1906 the new Local Education Authorities had the power to provide school meals for the needy, and in 1907 medical examination of schoolchildren was made compulsory. War had increased malnutrition, especially among children in the German and Austrian cities where severe forms of rickets became commonplace. Harriette Chick and her team of researchers went to Vienna in 1919, and found that sunlight, either natural or artificial, and cod-liver oil, to compensate for vitamin deficiencies, could both cure and prevent rickets. This knowledge of the social needs of children, both the sick and those most at risk, led the Hospital for Sick Children to propose, around 1920, a 'country hospital city for children'.

It was to be built about thirty miles from London, away from the smoke and dirt of the capital, and would consist of large groups of hospital pavilions with accommodation for staff and visiting parents. There, surrounded by trees, flowers and birds, sick children would flourish and grow strong in the sunshine and fresh air. The country hospital would cater for children from all over the world, not only from London. A small hospital and an out-patients department would be kept at Great Ormond Street. But only a fraction of the £2 million needed was ever raised. It was not an impossible and idealistic dream. Before the days of antibiotics such a country hospital seemed the only possible means of curing many of the crippling childhood diseases. Garden cities had already been built at Letchworth and Welwyn, and they still influence the ideals of town planners.

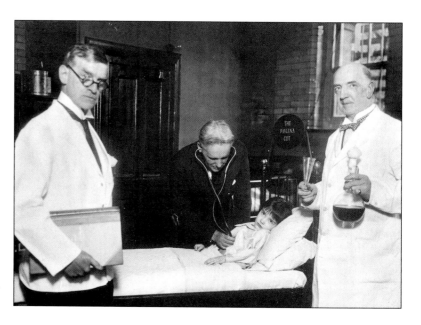

74 Dr Poynton carries out an examination. Mr McKay, hospital secretary (L), and Mr J. Wicliffe Peck, chief pharmacist (R), are also in attendance.

Tadworth Court

A country hospital for children was built at last, although on a much more modest scale, when Tadworth Court in Surrey was bought in 1927. The hospital's old convalescent home – seventeenth-century Cromwell House, Highgate – had after nearly half a century of use become impractical to maintain and was sold in 1924. At Tadworth, in the large and beautiful park of the Queen Anne mansion not far from Reigate, a pavilion for patients was opened in 1932 by the Prince of Wales (the hospital's president since 1919), the first of several pavilions to be built over the years.

The hospital was now receiving patients from all over the world. In 1924 an Indian Army regiment collected funds

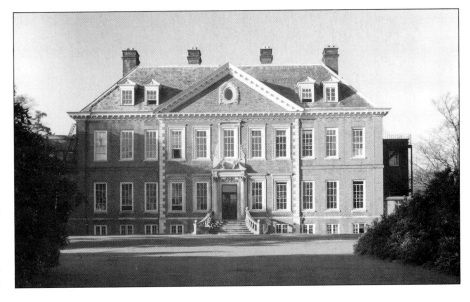

ABOVE RIGHT: *75 Tadworth Court; the mansion.*

BELOW: *76 In the grounds of Tadworth Court, Surrey, pavilions were built for treatment and convalescence of children 'in the country air'.*

for their sergeant's two children to be sent to Great Ormond Street for a much-needed operation on their eyes. The children were very young, and had been used to sleeping together. When they came back from the operating theatre with heavily bandaged eyes they were put in separate cots, and protested loudly. But when they were placed together in one bed they lay quietly, holding each other's hands tightly for all the days before their bandages were removed and their sight restored.

But there was still an urgent need for treatment for the poor children of London. A reporter visiting the hospital in 1925 described a little girl 'decorated now with pink ribbon of which she is now very proud, who had never slept upon a bed until she came to the

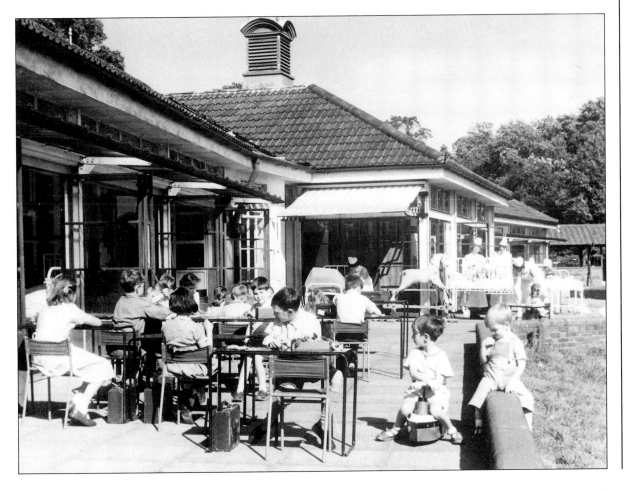

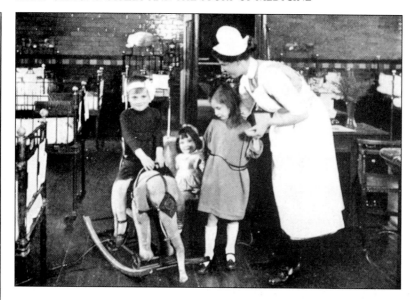

77 A scene in one of the wards in 1921. At this time there were nine wards with fourteen to twenty-seven beds in each. In total there were 244 beds.

Hospital'. She lived with her out-of-work father, her mother and brothers and sisters in one room, and had always had to sleep on a chair, so that her spine was badly affected. The reporter then described the rather run-down state of some of the wards, and expressed the hope that J. M. Barrie's Peter Pan 'could fly in at the window and paint these walls himself'. Four years later this wish was to come true.

Plans to rebuild

When the nearby Foundling Hospital decided to move to the country in 1929, many thought that was a wonderful opportunity for Great Ormond Street to rebuild on the tree-lined nine-acre open site. Great Ormond Street, although looked upon as a leader in the field of paediatric medicine, was housed in an out-of-date building with inadequate facilities, which compared very unfavourably with the splendid new children's hospitals in Europe and America, and even those in other British cities. When the third International Paediatric Congress was held in London in 1933, Great Ormond Street's Dr Still was president by virtue of being professor of children's diseases at King's College Hospital, London. Sir Thomas Barlow, at 88 the doyen of all the children's doctors present, received a tremendous ovation after speaking. But going round the hospital later many delegates were amazed that a new building had not been provided long before and that the

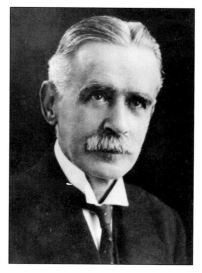

78 Sir George Frederic Still, consulting physician to the hospital. Reputedly the first paediatrician in Britain in that he devoted all his time to treating children.

staff were expected to work in such old-fashioned and cramped conditions. Fifty years later Great Ormond Street staff heard visiting doctors from abroad saying almost the same about the Southwood Building which was opened so proudly in 1938. The inexorable advance and demands of modern medicine seem almost always one step ahead of the hospital builders.

J. M. Barrie and Peter Pan

In February 1929 the hospital formed a fundraising committee in an attempt to buy the Foundling site. Among the eminent people they approached was J. M. Barrie, whose children's play *Peter Pan* had been performed every Christmas since 1904. In his reply, Barrie refused to serve on the committee, but thought he might find another way of helping the hospital.

It was not realised then, nor even today, that he had already known the hospital for many years. When he came to London in 1885, his first lodgings were very near Great Ormond Street, and it was in this house, at the corner of Greville Street, that he later placed the Darlings' nursery in *Peter Pan*. Every day Barrie walked along Guilford Street, and from here he could see the hospital's garden, where the children sat in wheelchairs around the Wishing Well fountain or played their first hesitant games when they grew stronger. He could not know that his name and Peter Pan's would become associated for ever with the children of Great Ormond Street. Barrie's first officially recorded donation was in 1908. His friend the Earl of Wemyss was chairman of Great Ormond Street from 1922 to 1927, and the Earl's daughter, Lady Cynthia Asquith, was Barrie's secretary from 1918 to 1937.

It was in April 1929 that Barrie gave Great Ormond Street *Peter Pan*, all royalties and rights to take effect immediately. It was an amazingly generous and unexpected gift. At Barrie's own request the amount raised by *Peter Pan* is never to be revealed, but apart from becoming

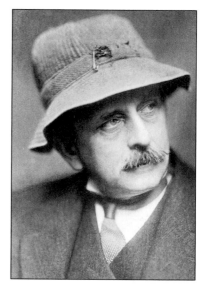

79 Sir James Barrie, author of Peter Pan.

80 Children and their nurses around the 'wishing well' fountain in the garden of the hospital in 1905.

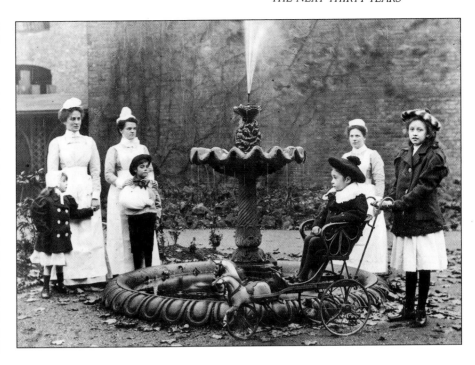

the most munificent gift ever given to the hospital, Peter Pan became a symbol and champion of children in hospital everywhere. A. A. Milne, another famous children's author, used his own characters of Christopher Robin and Winnie-the-Pooh in a brochure launching the Peter Pan League which encouraged children to support the work of the hospital. Children in Britain and North America eagerly joined. In December 1929, at Barrie's suggestion, the London cast of *Peter Pan* came to Great Ormond Street and performed the nursery scene in one of the wards. The famous actress Jean Forbes-Robertson, who played Peter Pan, remembered: 'The reception we received from the children will always live in my mind as a truly treasured moment.'

In the end Lord Rothermere decided to preserve the Foundling Hospital site intact as an open space for the benefit of local children and residents. As a result we have today Coram's Fields, one of the best playgrounds for children in London. The hospital could not quarrel with this decision but it was, nevertheless, a blow to Great Ormond Street's hopes and plans. Something of the bitter disappointment felt by the hospital can be seen on the cover of the thick file of papers dealing with the Foundling site, on which the hospital's secretary, James McKay, scrawled 'R.I.P.', after receiving Lord Rothermere's letter of refusal dated 27 June 1929.

The new hospital building

It was decided after all to reconstruct the hospital on its original Great Ormond Street site. As a first step a new nurses' home, facing Guilford Street, was opened in 1934 and an extension to it in 1937. Then the new hospital building was opened in October 1938 when King George VI and Queen Elizabeth visited Great Ormond Street. In those days before the introduction of antibiotics, each ward was designed to hold only ten children, including four separate cubicles, intended mainly for infants. This was to control the spread of gastro-intestinal and respiratory infections to which infants were so liable in the larger wards of the old hospital. For example, pioneer work has been done at Great Ormond Street on the treatment of

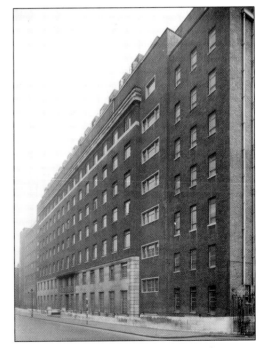

ABOVE: *81 The Princess Royal Nurses' Home, named after HRH Princess Mary, president of the hospital. The design for this building received the medal of the Royal Institute of British Architects.*

LEFT: *82 Actress Jean Forbes-Robertson and the cast of* Peter Pan *performing in Helena Ward in December 1929.*

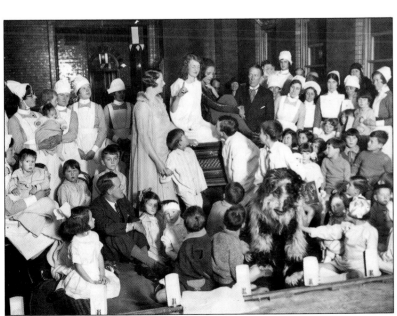

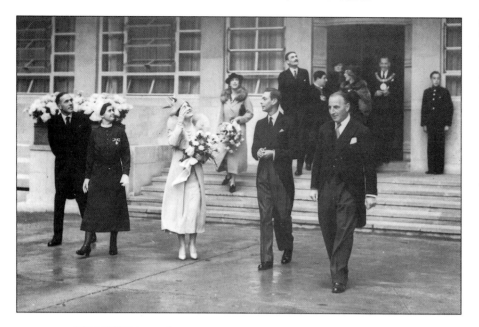

83 Their Majesties King George VI and Queen Elizabeth visit the hospital on 18 October 1938.

infants suffering from pyloric stenosis, a constriction of part of the stomach which required an operation. In the old hospital the mortality rate, mostly from post-operative infection, was between fifteen and twenty per cent year after year (in 1925, forty-nine of these operations were performed and eleven babies died). In the new 1938 wards, mortality fell to one or two per cent; when antibiotics became available after the Second World War, hundreds of such operations took place without one infant dying.

The new building, which was not named for Lord Southwood, the hospital's chairman, until after his death in 1946, meant that the hospital now had 326 beds, including 36 for private patients. Tadworth Court had a further 117 beds. Plans for further reconstruction, especially of the out-patients department, were stopped by the outbreak of the Second World War.

The Second World War

During the first eight months of 1939, 5,060 children were admitted as in-patients and 77,573 as out-patients. When the Second World War started at the beginning of September, the children with their doctors and nurses were evacuated to country hospitals at Hemel Hempstead, Haywards Heath, Watford, and, of course, Tadworth. Great Ormond Street became an emergency medical station with seventy-five beds for adult and child air-raid casualties. It had what was reputed to be the best-equipped and safest emergency operating theatre in London, built in the basement of the partially constructed new out-patients building. The hospital's senior physician, Dr Robert Frew, and its

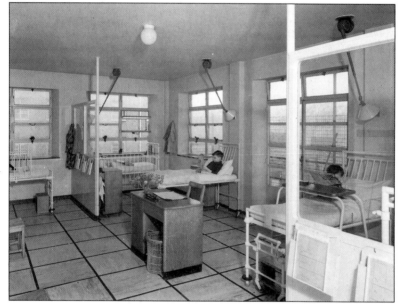

CENTRE: 84 The ward block opened in 1937 contained small wards of six beds as well as cubicles for individual patients.

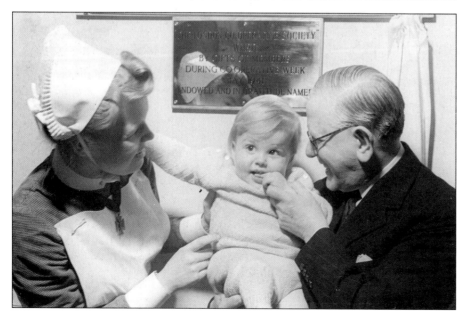

BOTTOM: 85 Lord Southwood, chairman of the hospital and a great benefactor, is seen here with a young patient.

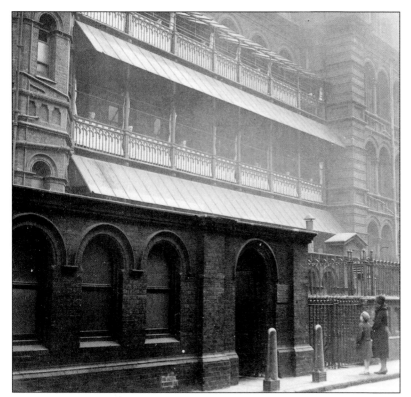

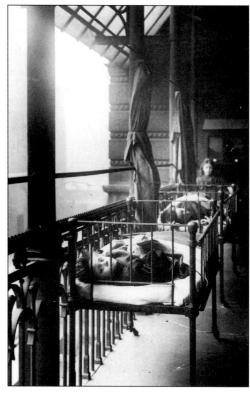

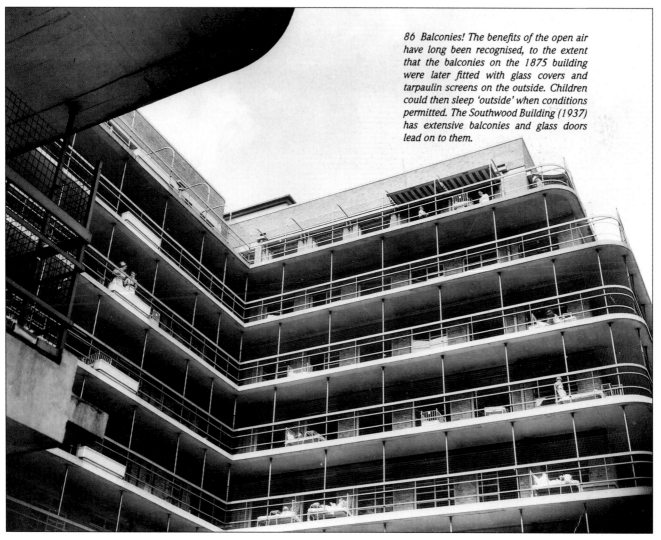

86 Balconies! The benefits of the open air have long been recognised, to the extent that the balconies on the 1875 building were later fitted with glass covers and tarpaulin screens on the outside. Children could then sleep 'outside' when conditions permitted. The Southwood Building (1937) has extensive balconies and glass doors lead on to them.

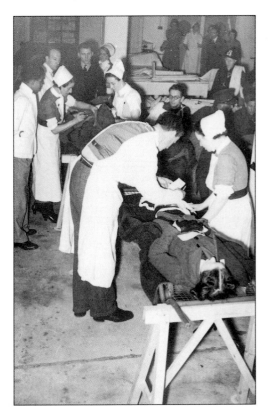

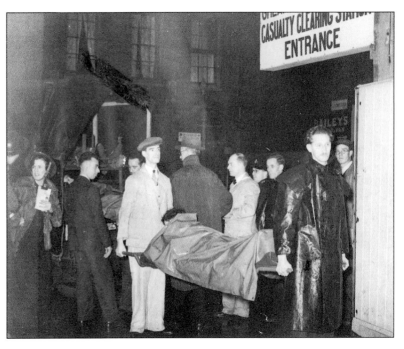

87 Second World War, 1939–45. The hospital acted as a casualty clearing station, admitting adult patients for the one and only time in its history. An operating theatre was installed in the basement of the partially constructed out-patients department, which had been started in 1938 but was not finished until long after the war.

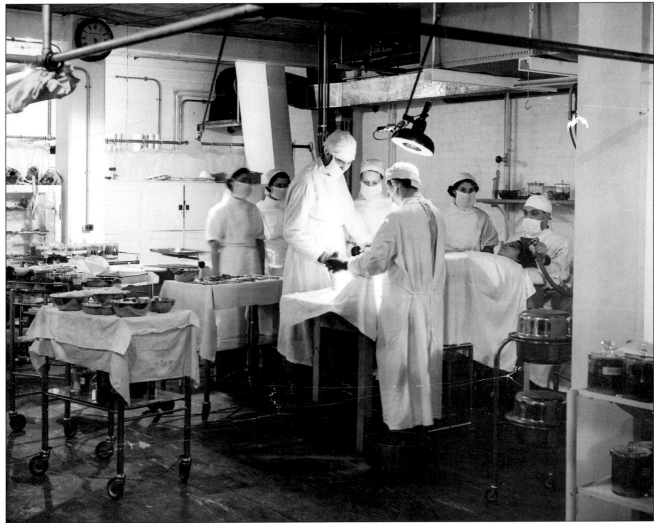

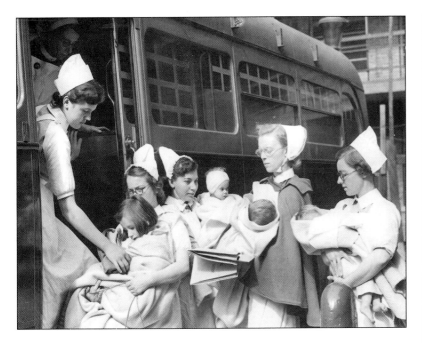

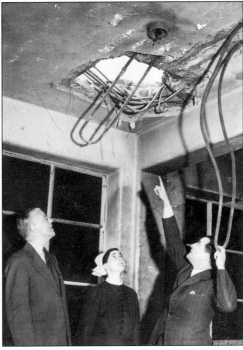

surgeons Sir Denis Browne and James Crooks, took charge of this casualty clearing station.

Throughout the war a few beds for children needing urgent treatment and an out-patients department were kept at Great Ormond Street. The hospital was bombed and damaged in September 1940. Part of a ward was destroyed and other wards had walls and ceilings

ABOVE LEFT: *88 Evacuation of children from the hospital at the outbreak of the Second World War (1939–45).*

ABOVE: *89 In September 1940 a stick of bombs straddled Great Ormond Street and Guilford Street. Damage was done to the Southwood Building but no one was injured. Miss Lane, the matron, and Mr H. Rutherford, the house governor (R), survey the damage.*

damaged, but children and staff had already moved to a shelter and nobody was hurt. As the threat of bombing lessened, more children were admitted and treated in the hospital. A boy who was in Great Ormond Street for an operation when the war ended remembered the nurses taking turns to join in the celebrations outside, coming back with flags for the children. His most vivid memory was of the house surgeons bursting triumphantly into the ward, laughing, dishevelled and dusty, having just knocked down the brick blast wall which had provided protection from exploding bombs and had stood outside the hospital door for nearly six years.

TIME CHART

AD

1887 Edison and Swan produce first domestic electric lamp.
1888 Hertz identifies wireless waves.
1890 London School Board appoints medical officer for schoolchildren.
1899–1901 Boer War.
1901 Marconi transmits Morse wireless signals across Atlantic.
1903 Wright brothers make first flight in heavier-than-air machine.
1904 *Peter Pan* first performed.
1906 Medical examination of schoolchildren compulsory. Rutherford deduces existence of atomic nucleus.
1908 Ford produces first cheap motor car, the Model T Ford.
1914–18 First World War. First women on medical staff of Great Ormond Street.
1918–19 Influenza epidemic causes nearly twenty million deaths.
1919 Dame Harriette Chick researches diet deficiencies and rickets in Vienna. Ministry of Health replaces local government boards.

1920 Great Ormond Street unsuccessfully propose 'country hospital city for children'. First public wireless broadcasting stations open in England and USA.
1921 First birth control clinic opens in London.
1924 Cromwell House, Highgate, sold.
1927 Tadworth Court acquired as a country branch for Great Ormond Street.
1929 J. M. Barrie gives Great Ormond Street all rights to *Peter Pan*.
1932 First open-air pavilion opened at Tadworth by Prince of Wales.
1933 International Paediatric Congress held in London with Dr Still as president.
1934 New nurses' home opened in Guilford Street.
1938 New hospital building (later the Southwood Building) opened.
1939 Second World War begins. Patients evacuated to country. Great Ormond Street becomes an emergency casualty station.
1940 Great Ormond Street damaged by bombs.
1945 Second World War ends.

CHAPTER 7

Medicine and Science 1919–42

Advances in surgery

It was during the First World War that blood storage was first attempted, with some limited success. After the war, hospitals reverted to the practice of using an individual donor for each transfusion. It was not until the Spanish Civil War of 1936–9 that blood storage was again tried. Blood banks were then fully developed during the Second World War.

Another aspect of medicine which advanced in both world wars was plastic surgery, first under Sir Harold Gillies,

90 Sir Denis Browne (1892–1967).

then under Sir Archibald McIndoe. After 1945 David Matthews enlarged the scope of plastic surgery at Great Ormond Street. For children who were disfigured by a congenital malformation, by accident or burns, plastic surgery not only restored their features or bodies to something approaching normality, but also provided a tremendous psychological boost, and changed an understandably withdrawn, apathetic child into an active, happy one. In recent years, plastic surgery has been an important part of the surgical attempt to correct grave abnormalities previously thought inoperable.

When Gasparo Tagliacozzi of Bologna pioneered plastic surgery at the end of the sixteenth century, he was criticised for daring to meddle with the handiwork of God. So strong was the opposition he aroused that his body was exhumed from the convent where it lay and reburied in unconsecrated ground. Plastic surgery then fell into disrepute and disuse until it was revived by German surgeons in 1816, the year Charles West was born. The modern method of skin-grafting was first used by Karl Thiersch of Leipzig in 1874.

At Great Ormond Street, the most important contribution to the development of paediatric surgery after 1918 was made by Sir Denis Browne. He arrived at the hospital in 1922, and as Sir Frederic Still was the first to confine himself to paediatric medicine, so Denis Browne was the first to confine his work to children's surgery. He pioneered surgery on the newborn (neonatal surgery), and was the first surgeon there to make extended observations of congenital abnormalities. He improved orthopaedic surgery, especially in the treatment of talipes (club-foot). Like all great men, he

had his eccentricities. When the cleaners kept shifting his office chair from its exact favoured position, he screwed it to the wall. He was sometimes brusque, obstinate and impatient. Like Charles West, who had the reputation of being a difficult man to work with, Browne could be at loggerheads with his professional colleagues in London and elsewhere; but like West he had many devoted admirers, and children and parents immediately responded to him. In the two decades after the war there were enormous developments in paediatric surgery and cardiac surgery and his career extended into these years. Typically, he had been operating only two weeks before he died in January 1967, aged 74. Sir David Innes Williams, who worked with him at Great Ormond Street, described him as 'in every way a remarkable character . . . looking back no-one can deny the enormous impact of his personality on Great Ormond Street or on the evolution of paediatric surgery'.

Much of this advance was made possible through improvements in anaesthetics and their administration. One problem, which was to continue for decades, was how to avoid causing frightened children distress when they were being anaesthetized. Harold Sington, the hospital's first honorary consultant anaesthetist, was appointed in 1908. He was troubled by the sight of children about to have their tonsils removed, being separated from their mothers in the out-patients department and taken, screaming with fright, to the adjoining operating theatre. There, the terrified child often had to be held down by the out-patient sister and porter while chloroform was dripped on to a gauze mask. This procedure, as the present writer experienced, was still much the same at Queen Elizabeth Hospital for Children around 1930. Sington introduced.the idea of 'premedication', where the patient was sedated before the operation. Unfortunately, the one drug which was then at all suitable for children was paraldehyde. This required rectal administration to children lying in their cots, something which many children disliked. Nevertheless, the ideal of sensitive pre-operative care started in Great Ormond Street, and influenced other hospitals.

Yet as late as 1953, a surgeon wrote in *The Lancet,* 'the premedication of chil-

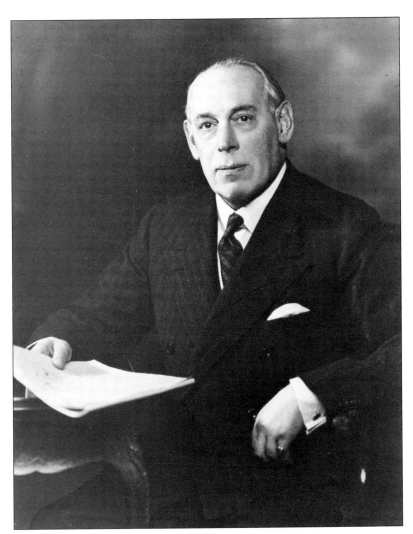

The discovery of insulin

One of the most important results of earlier work on hormones and enzymes was the discovery and isolation of insulin in 1921. Millions of people suffering from diabetes can now lead ordinary lives without fear of blindness or gangrene or an early death in coma. Diabetes mellitus was probably known as long ago as Ancient Egypt; the Ebers papyrus gave a prescription against the passing of too much urine. In Roman times, Celsius described a similar condition associated with hunger, thirst and emaciation. Around AD 100 Aretaeus of Cappadocia first named it 'diabetes' after the Greek for 'I go through', describing its symptoms and the short life of the sufferer. Rhazes, Avicenna and Paracelsus all made observations on the disease. Thomas Willis of Oxford first fully described the sweet taste of diabetic urine in the seventeenth century, but it had been noted in Ancient India two thousand years before. In France around the time of the Battle of Waterloo, Chevreul identified this sugar with glucose, and Claude Bernard's work a generation later on the production of glucose by the liver gave the real impetus for research into diabetes.

In 1923 Dr Poynton described the fate of five cases of diabetes mellitus in one ward at Great Ormond Street, shortly before treatment with insulin became generally available. Poynton said that while the disease was fortunately not common in childhood, it is then that 'we see the pure type of virulent diabetes'. Three boys and two girls, aged between 5 and 9, were his patients. 'We had all, according to our lights, worked most diligently at them; yet all died within three years.' Their main treatment was a controlled diet which, as Poynton realised, 'only touched the fringe of the problem'. The children had been in and out of hospital as they seemed to recover and then broke down again, which added to their distress. In the last terminal stages of the disease one girl 'became very unhappy . . . at her urgent request she went home, dying in a coma in November 1922'.

dren is one of the most important unsolved problems in modern anaesthetics . . . For any child to go conscious to the anaesthetic room smacks of the surgical Middle Ages.' B. G. B. Lucas, then Great Ormond Street's anaesthetist, also expressed doubts about the effectiveness of sedatives on children, as they could produce a nightmare state of semi-drowsiness: 'Children should reach the anaesthetic room prior to surgery either fast asleep or in complete possession of their faculties.' With better drugs children and adults are now spared this unnecessary trauma.

Modern anaesthesia began when quick-acting barbiturates were found in the 1930s. Curare, the South American arrow poison, was purified, adapted and tested in 1942. Great Ormond Street was one of the first hospitals to use it with an anaesthetic, when a baby only twenty hours old with a very large umbilical hernia was operated on successfully and without complications. Curare, a muscle relaxant, and other

similar drugs made long and complicated neonatal and cardiac surgery possible, without any of the former time risk.

Major surgery of the heart and of the large blood vessels began in the early 1940s. Just at this time, Alexis Carrel, who had won a Nobel Prize in 1912 for his work on vascular suture and the transplantation of veins and organs, died in disgrace after the liberation of Paris. He was accused of collaborating with the Germans. During 1914–18, together with the English surgeon D. H. Dakin, he had developed the Carrel–Dakin solution for the treatment of deep wounds, which prevented infection and had saved many lives on the battlefield. Without his pioneer work none of the more spectacular advances in modern surgery would have been possible. In 1935 he had invented a form of mechanical heart, a perfusion pump which kept whole organs alive in his laboratory with a supply of artificial blood. It was not until 1952 that a heart-lung machine was used in cardiac surgery.

'A great step forward'

Poynton hoped that insulin might produce very different results; if so, he wrote, 'a great step forward has been made in medical knowledge'. Paul Langerhans at Berlin in 1869, and Joseph von Mering and Oscar Minkowski at Strasbourg twenty years later, had shown that a deficiency in the pancreas caused diabetes. The long search for the active principle of the 'islets of Langerhans' ended with the discoveries of Frederick Grant Banting and Charles Best at Professor John Macleod's laboratory at Toronto, where earlier Banting had been an orthopaedic surgeon at its Hospital for Sick Children.

After the insulin had been isolated and tested it was administered to a 14-year-old boy who had been a diabetic for two years. When he was admitted to the Toronto General Hospital in January 1922, he was emaciated and distressed, just like the children Poynton with growing and helpless despair was watching die in his ward at Great Ormond Street. But the Toronto boy was saved. In 1921, forty per cent of all diabetic patients died in a coma; by 1975, the figure was only a fraction of one per cent.

In 1924 Great Ormond Street asked for free supplies of insulin from the Ministry of Health, but was told that no funds were available for this purpose. It is said that the hospital was one of the first to manufacture its own insulin, using pancreases from the slaughterhouse at the Caledonian Market. Research continued. In 1926 John Abel of Baltimore synthesized insulin in a crystalline form. In 1945 Frederick Sanger and Dorothy Hodgkin began eight years' research. Using the technique of X-ray diffraction, they determined the structure of the amino acids – the basic constituents of protein – in the insulin molecule. The same X-ray technique played an important part in the epoch-making discovery of the genetic code by Watson, Crick, Khorana and others. Perhaps in the future, genetic engineering will be able to correct the inborn error of metabolism which causes diabetes.

Vitamins and children's diseases

In 1926 G. R. Minot and W. P. Murphy began the successful treatment of pernicious anaemia with liver, and later a liver extract was used. The isolation of Vitamin B12 in 1948 provided an even more powerful cure for this deficiency disease.

During the years between the wars, there was much useful work done on vitamins. In the 1920s Joseph Goldberger showed that pellagra, a deficiency disease causing dermatitis and often leading to madness, could be prevented by Vitamin B. The isolation of Vitamin C as ascorbic acid was achieved by W. A. Waugh and C. G. King in 1932. Two years later it was synthesized by W. N. Haworth at Birmingham. In California, H. M. Evans culminated his work on Vitamin E by isolating it from wheat germ in 1936. Vitamin A was obtained in its pure crystalline form by H. A. Homes and Ruth Corbet in 1937, and synthesized during the war. All this research into vitamins was to be of great value in the study of children's diseases, and work is still continuing. One example within the last few years is the Institute of Child Health's investigation of the role of Vitamin E in the neurological function of children with chronic and severe disorders of fat malabsorption, undertaken in collaboration with other hospitals in London and researchers in the USA and Canada.

When it appeared in 1939, DDT was the most powerful insecticide yet known. It controlled threatened outbreaks of louse-borne typhus during and after the war, and cleared the tsetse-fly, the carrier of sleeping sickness, from many areas. The World Health Organization encouraged its use in mosquito elimination. Although at one time seemingly successful, the control of mos-

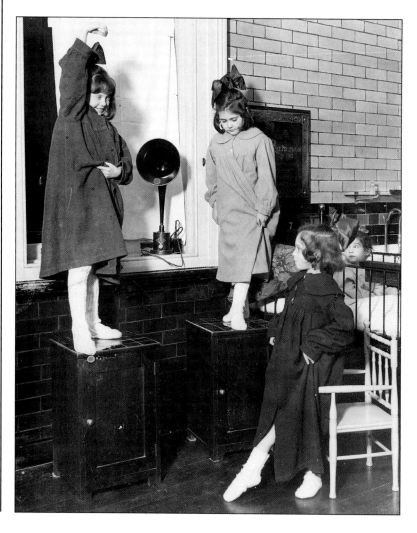

92 In 1922 the British Broadcasting Corporation installed ten loudspeakers in the hospital to receive programmes from their new broadcasting station. These convalescent patients are evidently enjoying a music programme.

quitoes has not been effective and malaria is now making a serious come-back in Africa and elsewhere. It soon appeared that DDT had a grave disadvantage – mosquitoes and other disease-carrying insects developed an in-built resistance to the insecticide. It has also persistent toxicity which spreads through the food-chain of insects, birds, animals and man. Strict controls on its use were imposed, but these were not always effective, and researchers developed replacement drugs. The fact that yellow fever no longer poses a serious threat, despite failure to eliminate the mosquito, is due to the vaccine against it, which was first found in 1932, and later improved. Yellow fever is a virus disease. Further profitable study of virus-caused diseases had to wait for the electron microscope and the radioisotope. But vastly improved remedies for bacterial disease and infection had already been found before 1939 and were soon to be perfected.

A miraculous remedy

Ehrlich's Salvarsan worked against the micro-organisms, the spirochaetes, which cause syphilis. For a long time quinine had been a remedy against the protozeal parasites of malaria. During the First World War the Germans became worried about obtaining their supplies of quinine from the Dutch East Indies, and began trying to find a chemical substitute, following the lead of Ehrlich's earlier work with aniline dyes. Ehrlich died in 1915, and it was not until 1933, after testing 12,000 compounds, that Mepacrine was developed, then the most effective anti-malarial drug. But still no chemotherapeutical remedy had been found against cocci and bacilli, the sphere-shaped and straight rod-shaped bacteria which cause many of the commoner, but potentially dangerous, infections outside the tropics. At the same Elberfeld laboratories, and working with the same research team which had discovered Mepacrine, Gerhard Domagk began experimenting with a new synthetic dye, prontosil red. Although this appeared inert in the test-tube, it halted the process of septicaemia when tested on mice – it worked only in the living organism.

In 1935 Domagk's young daughter,

Hildegarde, developed severe blood poisoning after pricking her finger with a knitting needle and accidentally handling a culture of bacteria in her father's laboratory. Domagk, afraid that she might die, gave her Prontosil. The hitherto inexorable septicaemia was halted, and Hildegarde recovered. Domagk was overjoyed. He had not only saved his daughter with the first test on a human of an untried remedy, when the desperate concern of a father had overcome his scientific caution, but he had also discovered one of the miraculous remedies of modern medicine.

After Domagk's paper on Prontosil was published later that year, the Medical Research Council in London asked Dr Leonard Colebrook to make one of the first clinical trials of the new drug at Queen Charlotte's Maternity Hospital. In the previous 50 years 100,000 mothers had died of puerperal fever in England and Wales, even after Pasteur and Lister had shown the true cause of infections. It was no mere whimsy that made J. M. Barrie write in 1902: 'The only ghosts . . . are dead young mothers, returned to see how their children fare.' Dr Colebrook's tests found that Prontosil drastically reduced the mortality from puerperal fever (known to the Victorians as childbed fever) to a mere fraction of its

previous rate. This, as Dr Colebrook said, had never been seen before in his ten years' experience at Queen Charlotte's Hospital.

Not long after this, the Pasteur Institute in Paris found that the active antibacterial element in Prontosil was one of a group of sulphonamide drugs. A whole new series of healing drugs was derived from this discovery. One of the most famous was M & B 693, found by Ewins and Phillips in 1938, which saved Winston Churchill when he became seriously ill with pneumonia in North Africa during the war. By then Fleming's earlier discovery of penicillin was being mass produced in America, and the antibiotics were to prove an even more powerful weapon against infection than the sulphonamides.

Alexander Fleming and penicillin

Bacteriologists had observed since the time of Pasteur that certain micro-organisms normally present in the soil

93 Sir Alexander Fleming (1881–1955), discoverer of penicillin.

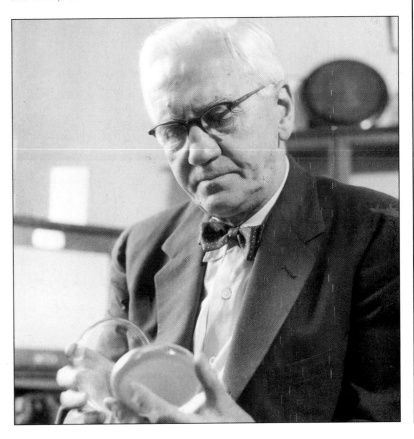

sometimes inhibit the growth of other micro-organisms. This antagonism between one bacterium and another was called 'antibiosis'. In 1928 at St Mary's Hospital, London, Alexander Fleming discovered penicillin after noticing that a mould which had contaminated a culture of common staphylococcus, often the origin of wound infections and boils, had begun to destroy the microbes. From this chance observation came the most important contribution to medicine in the twentieth century – antibiotics.

Fleming published his first report on penicillin in 1929. An old pupil of his, Dr C. G. Paine in Sheffield, took some filtered liquid Fleming had prepared from the penicillin and used it on four newborn babies, whose eyes were full of pus from gonococcal conjunctivitis, which usually causes permanent damage to the sight and blindness. Within a few days, the eyes of three of the babies were clear

94 Sir Alexander Fleming's laboratory in St Mary's Hospital, Paddington.

of pus and infection. This was the first clinical demonstration of penicillin's remarkable powers. As Fleming later noted, it was 'not interfered with by the presence of blood as was that of many of the older antiseptics, and unlike the sulphonamides, its action was maintained in pus'. But Fleming lacked a full research team of specialists, and the complicated chemical problems of making penicillin remained unsolved for ten years. It was only then that its full possibilities and remarkable qualities were fully realised.

At Oxford in 1938, Professor Howard Florey and Dr Ernst Chain, who had been working together on Fleming's earlier discovery of lysozyme, which is one of the body's natural defences against bacteria, decided to follow this up with an investigation into penicillin. Since Fleming's paper of 1929 only one attempt had been made to purify it, an unsuccessful experiment at the London School of Hygiene and Tropical Medicine in 1932. Florey and Chain, together with

Dr Heatley and Professor Gardner, assembled a group of bacteriologists, pathologists, chemists, surgeons, doctors and technicians, all of whom were to be needed for the task of purifying and concentrating the penicillin to realise its full potentialities and test it in the laboratory and finally on the human subject. Even so, producing sufficient penicillin was always one of the main problems. In fact all this early work at Oxford was done with penicillin directly descended from Fleming's original mould. The brownish powder they eventually produced and worked with was crude compared with the refined white penicillin which was afterwards manufactured. A vial of this vital Oxford mould was later to be carefully carried all the way to America.

The first patient, a policeman desperately ill with rapidly spreading blood poisoning against which even the sulphonamide drugs seemed helpless, was given penicillin in 1941. His condition improved considerably, then the supplies

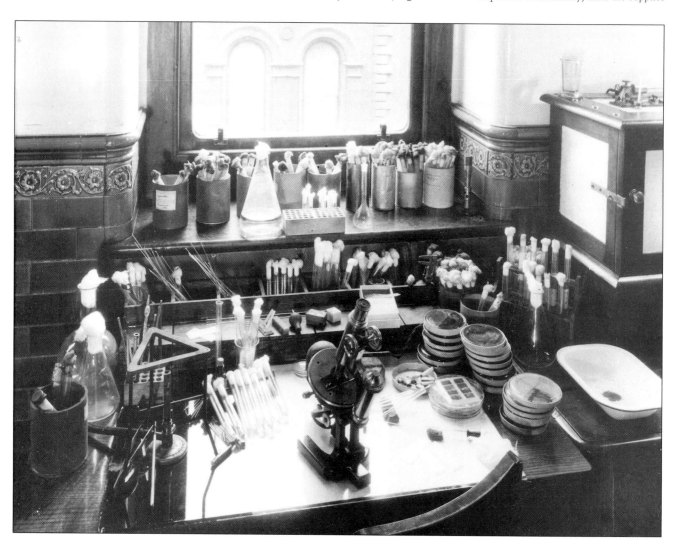

of penicillin ran out and in the few days before fresh supplies could be prepared the infection returned, and the patient died. Now everyone knew that penicillin must be administered without pause for at least several days. A 15-year-old boy with a very dangerous post-operative infection of the hip was near death. With penicillin which was recovered from the urine of the first patient, the boy, against all previous medical precedent, was completely cleared of infection. His was the first human life to be saved by penicillin. Several further cases of severe infection were treated with complete success.

New hope from America

At that time the war was raging in Europe. Scientists knew that the miraculous healing powers of penicillin would be a godsend in treating casualties on the battlefields. The only hope for the mass production of a purified penicillin was in America. The Rockefeller Foundation which had originally supported the Oxford series of tests (the few hundred pounds awarded was surely one of the most worthwhile research grants ever made) invited Dr Florey to go to America. Although production on a small but useful scale did start in Britain, 300 million units a month in 1943, it was in America that production began on a massive scale where over £5 million was spent on factories and equipment by the end of 1943. America was then producing over 9,000 million units of penicillin each month. By the end of the war, in August 1945, 800,000 million units flowed from the factories each month. The total number of lives saved then and since are countless.

Penicillin has a bactericidal action: it kills the bacteria outright, whereas other antibiotics, like streptomycin and aureomycin, are bacteriostatic – they inhibit and prevent the growth of bacteria. Sulphonamides also halt the growth of bacteria by interfering with their metabolism, whereupon they are more easily attacked and eliminated by the phagocytes in the bloodstream.

Penicillin, like all antibiotics and chemotherapy, can be abused. It was such an easy and effective cure that in the early days there was a tendency to prescribe it for the mildest of infections. Penicillin-sensitive patients were found allergic to it. Bacteria began to develop drug-resistant strains. The appearance of such drug-resistant infections was first noted around 1948, and this became a major problem, especially in hospitals. The development of other and newer forms of penicillin, especially of synthetic penicillin, overcame some of these difficulties. The benefit to humanity, however, enormously outweighed any possible drawbacks.

There had already been an unexplained natural decrease in certain childhood illnesses and infections. No doubt, the better care of babies and children, the commercial refrigeration of food and the pasteurisation of milk, improved sanitation, better housing and living conditions and more effective immunisation had all helped. Infantile diarrhoea, dysentery, infections of the ear, nose and throat and the skin, the rheumatic diseases, had all become much less common. The story of the decline of tuberculosis and poliomyelitis is told in Chapter 9.

But apart from all this, there is no question that the sulphonamides and the antibiotics have considerably reduced the number of deaths from once common childhood infections, and helped to decrease their incidence. This is shown in the admissions to children's hospitals everywhere.

TIME CHART

AD
1597 Gasparo Tagliacozzi pioneers plastic surgery.
1816 C. F. von Graefe founds modern plastic surgery.
1874 Karl Thiersch improves skin-grafting.
c. 1908 Sington introduces premedication for children at Great Ormond Street.
1912 Alexis Carrel wins Nobel Prize for work on suturing veins and transplanting blood-vessels and organs.
1914–22 Sir Harold Gillies improves plastic surgery for disfigured and wounded soldiers.
1914–18 Carrel and Dakin develop Carrel–Dakin solution for treatment of deep wounds.
1915 Tetanus anti-toxin successfully given to wounded.
1916 Blood stored under refrigeration for transfusion.
1922 F. Banting and C. H. Best isolate insulin and administer it to a diabetic boy. Sir Denis Browne develops paediatric surgery and pioneers neonatal surgery at Great Ormond Street.
c. 1923 J. Goldberger treats pellagra with Vitamin B.
c. 1924 Great Ormond Street begins to manufacture its own supplies of insulin.
1926 G. R. Minot and W. P. Murphy treat pernicious anaemia with liver.
1928–9 Sir Alexander Fleming discovers penicillin.
1932 Waugh and King isolate Vitamin C as ascorbic acid. Vaccine against yellow fever developed.
1933 Mepacine developed as anti-malarial drug.
1935 Gerhard Domagk discovers Prontosil, the first sulphonamide drug. Carrel invents a form of mechanical heart.

1936 H. M. Evans isolates Vitamin E.
1936–7 H. N. Holmes and Ruth Corbet obtain pure crystalline Vitamin A.
1938 Ewins and Phillips develop M & B 693 against pneumonia.
1939 Paul Müller discovers DDT.
1939–41 Howard Florey and Ernst Chain investigate and develop penicillin.
c. 1940 Blood banks and blood plasma stored for transfusion.
1940 Sir Archibald McIndoe greatly improves plastic surgery of burnt and disfigured airmen. Major surgery of heart and large blood-vessels begins.
1942 Curare-derived drugs used as muscle relaxants in surgery.
1943 Mass production of penicillin begins in USA.
1944 C. T. Avery and others discover DNA, the nucleic acid.
1945 David Matthews enlarges scope of plastic surgery at Great Ormond Street.
1945–53 F. Sanger and Dorothy Hodgkin work on atomic structure of amino acids in insulin molecule.
1948 Smith and Rickes isolate anti-pernicious anaemia factor in liver, named B_{12}.
1950–60 Pincus, Rock and Chang develop birth control pill.
1952 Heart–lung machine first used in cardiac surgery.
1953 Watson, Crick and Wilkins discover double helix structure of DNA forming genetic code.
1968 H. G. Khorana shares Nobel Prize for work on deciphering the genetic code.

CHAPTER 8

Great Ormond Street from 1945

In 1922 the Board's Annual Report declared: 'The Institution of an adequate and purposely equipped Research Department for the study of the causes and treatment of children's diseases is highly desirable.' This was, of course, one of Charles West's aims when he founded the hospital. In 1942, in the middle of a world war, the first steps were taken in forming what was to become the Institute of Child Health. That year fierce battles raged in Russia, the Pacific and North Africa; Europe was being bombed day and night; and preparations were going ahead for building the first atomic bomb. It needed a remarkable degree of optimism and fore-sight to start planning an institute for paediatric research; but 1942 was also the year of the Beveridge Report, and a welfare state with a national health service suddenly seemed possible.

The Nuffield Foundation endowed a chair of child health at the University of London; Dr Alan Moncrieff, for many years on the staff at Great Ormond Street, became its first professor in 1945. The Institute of Child Health was opened the following year, using converted ground-floor rooms at the hospital. Its present large and well-equipped building in Guilford Street, facing the greenery of Coram's Fields, was completed in 1965 after £430,000 was raised by public subscription, and formally opened by the Queen in 1966.

The hospital and the Institute jointly encourage and support advanced research to improve the care of sick children and initiate new and effective treatments. A number of other professorial posts in various branches of paediatric medicine and associated sciences have been added to the original chair of child health. Doctors, scientists and nurses, radiologists, therapists and other paramedical staff come from all over the world to the hospital and the Institute. Like the staff, many patients come from abroad – from over a hundred countries in recent years, making up seven per cent of all the children treated in Great Ormond Street.

Classrooms in hospital

The first regular school teachers started work among the children at Tadworth Court in 1946. The children there were long-stay patients: ortho-paedic cases or suffering from various forms of rheumatism, chorea, tuberculosis and poliomyelitis. Sir Wilfrid Sheldon, who attended the royal children, was the

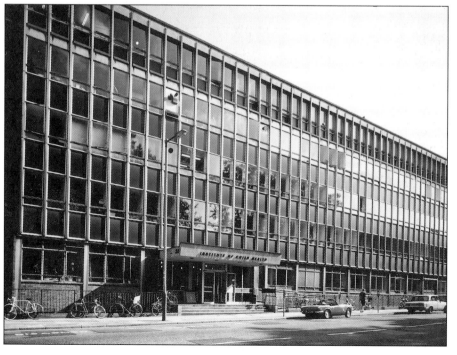

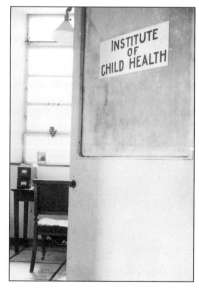

ABOVE: *95 Modest accommodation for the Institute of Child Health in the early days.*

LEFT: *96 The Institute of Child Health. Not only do the hospital and the Institute share a close functional relationship, but also they are close geographically, being on the same site between Great Ormond Street and Guilford Street.*

visiting physician at Tadworth when the school opened. Five years later Great Ormond Street also had a hospital school. Lessons were first given only in the wards, but classrooms were soon provided by what was then the Inner London Education Authority. Today, the London Borough of Camden is responsible.

As in all hospital schools, the teachers required great skill; they dealt not only with children of different ages and capabilities, but with children in various stages of severe illness and disability. The children produced work of a high standard, especially in their modelling and artwork, as they do today. Although some little boys were heard to say, 'School! What a swiz! I thought I'd get out of that here', the school offered a welcome relief from the routine and monotony of the ward. For those children not too ill to be taught, hospital school helped to restore confidence, a valuable first step on the road to recovery.

Today there are not so many long-stay children at Great Ormond Street, and most who remain for longer periods are very young. But about four years ago one of the few long-stay older children was helped with the preparations for his O-level examinations, which he took with great success when he returned to school after over a year's absence.

Teachers have altered their approach to meet changed conditions. Children now come from a much wider variety of cultural backgrounds than they did a generation ago. In the new school area, apart from a large classroom, a library and other facilities for staff and children, there is an up-to-date computer studies room. As many children as possible are brought to the classroom, which is also used by day patients at the neighbouring Haematology and Oncology Day Care Unit. Visits to places of interest in London are arranged as part of the hospital school's activities.

The hospital and the NHS

The organisation and funding of all hospitals changed dramatically when the National Health Service took over on 5 July 1948. The Government now paid within agreed limits for all running costs and salaries. Everybody, rich or poor, was entitled to treatment without charge. Consultants and senior physicians and surgeons were no longer honorary, but paid like all other staff, and no longer entirely dependent on private patients for a living. There has been much argument about the provision of private beds and clinics for paying patients on NHS premises, with implications of queue-jumping and other preferential treatment. At Great Ormond Street the admission of private patients has, on the whole, been beneficial to all the children. Private beds have helped to keep other wards and departments open when Government funding has been inadequate. Great Ormond Street became one of the eight postgraduate teaching hospitals. This meant the board of governors was directly responsible to the Ministry of Health, without any local or regional authority intervening. After further reorganisation of the NHS, the postgraduate hospitals each became their own Special Health Authority in 1982, exercising much the same functions in the same way. The board and the special trustees retain the use of their own endowment and trust funds for research, special equipment, improvements and other projects. Without these funds and continuing public support the work of the hospital would be severely restricted.

More access for mothers

The Hospital for Sick Children proudly celebrated its centenary in 1952, and the Queen visited the hospital that July. The Princess Royal, Mary, Countess of Harewood, who had trained as a nurse at Great Ormond Street during

97 HM The Queen visits the hospital in its centenary year, 1952. Miss G. M. Kirby, the matron, steps forward to greet her whilst the head porter, Mr J. Pusey, waits in attendance.

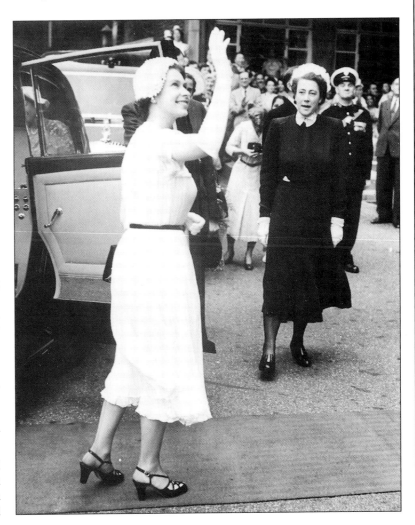

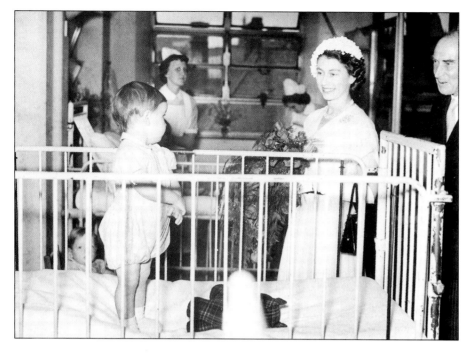

98 The Queen visits one of the wards. The considerable interest of many members of the Royal Family, from Queen Victoria onwards, has always been a great source of practical and moral support to patients, parents and staff.

the First World War and became a vice-patron in 1923 and president in 1936, laid the foundation stone of a new out-patients department. The old Astor Building had been demolished in 1938, and was never replaced because of building restrictions during and after the war.

In this centenary year the hospital took a great step forward in allowing mothers to see their children much more frequently. Visiting restrictions had already been quietly relaxed when the new Southwood Building was opened in 1938. After the war Professor Alan Moncrieff supported and influenced the growing movement across the country to give mothers more access to their children in hospital. In 1952 Great Ormond Street started the experiment of allowing mothers in every evening to visit their children, and tuck them up with a goodnight kiss after their usual bedtime story or chat. Other hospitals followed its example, particularly Northampton. Alan Moncrieff and Dr Mildred Creak, also of Great Ormond Street, were prominent members of a committee formed to advise on the whole question of parents and children in hospital. The Ministry of Health's 1959 Platt Report on the Welfare of Children in Hospital recommended unrestricted visiting for parents, finding that a mother staying with her child in hospital played an important role in the child's recovery, easing emotional problems and soothing fears. Now this is recognised and encouraged in hospitals all over the world. The Toronto Hospital for Sick Children, for example, involves the whole local community in the welfare of children in hospital.

Such names as James Spence, James Robertson, John Bowlby and Anna Freud

with their work at Newcastle, the Tavistock Clinic, the World Health Organization, and the Hampstead Child Therapy Clinic are usually cited as pioneers of the movement in this country. But Great Ormond Street in its early days had anticipated all this. A rule against admitting children under 2 was broken in the very first week of the hospital's existence, when a 14-month-old boy, Charles Cooper, became an in-patient on 20 February 1852. He was the first of many children under 2 to be admitted over the succeeding years. The rule was later altered; but in 1889 it still read that infants or children under 2 years of age would in special circumstances 'be received into the Hospital either *with or without their mothers*'. In the 1860s Wednesday was the parents' usual visiting day, but a dangerously ill child could be visited at any time of the day or night. Later, in 1882, an hour on Thursday and Sunday afternoons was allowed for normal visiting, but by 1893 only Sunday visiting was permitted. Visiting on Sundays only, between 2 p.m. and 3.30 p.m. was still the rule in 1916, and children under 14 could not visit the wards, a restriction in force for some time. This ban on children visiting the wards was general in nearly all hospitals until comparatively recently.

As confirmed in 1889, Great Ormond Street welcomed the general public every afternoon for visits of inspection, a method of attracting support and good publicity used from the hospital's beginning. Only in recent years did the Washington Children's Hospital arrange guided tours for the public. In Great Ormond Street's early days, younger children who were distressed when parents left the ward were always diverted within five minutes by the simple distraction of 'tea-time'. It was fear of infection, of the smuggling in of forbidden sweets and other foods, and perhaps a tendency to assume infallible authority on the part of certain doctors and highly efficient but overbearing ward sisters, which led to parents being regarded as a disturbing and upsetting presence in the wards, before Alan Moncrieff and others began to change things. On the whole,

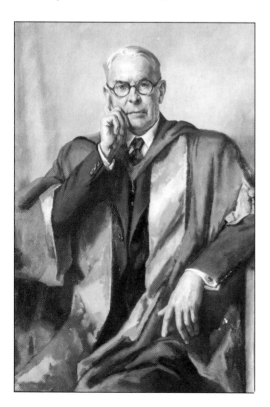

99 Professor Sir Alan Moncrieff (1901–71), first professor of child health in the Institute of Child Health, of which he was also director.

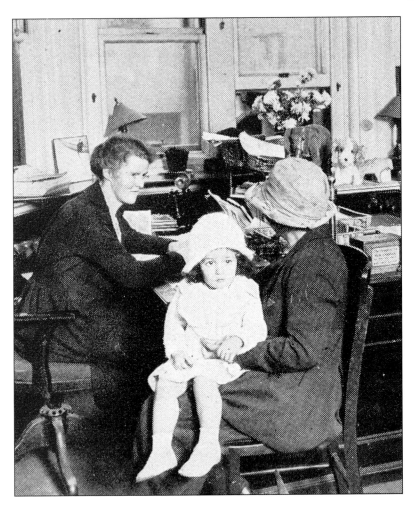

formations to be corrected after and sometimes even before birth. This meant a completely new cardiac wing was required. After various structural problems, the new wing became fully operational not long after the launch of the Wishing Well Appeal.

Since 1953 the hospital has sent medical and nursing staff to help child health services in Africa, the Middle East and other countries. A Tropical Child Health Unit at the Institute of Child Health trains and advises workers from developing countries and carries out research programmes in association with UNICEF and the WHO. Professor Moncrieff, who initiated this scheme, also developed community medicine in the hospital itself with the Province of Natal Centre for infant and child welfare. Exchanges of junior medical staff with the Philadelphia Children's Hospital and other hospitals for children have been very fruitful.

The new out-patients department was ready in 1954 (see page 68). Eight years later three storeys were added to the frontage for the Departments of Psychological Medicine, Physical Medicine and Medical Records. A Barrie Wing was opened with new X-ray and dental departments, and also a thoracic unit ward linked to the additional operating theatre which had already been added in 1959.

The training of nurses

The School of Nursing, later fittingly named after Charles West, moved to a new building in 1960. When the Queen Elizabeth Hospital for Children in Hackney Road joined the Hospitals for Sick Children Group it complemented the largely specialised work at Great Ormond Street and provided more comprehensive paediatric medical and nursing training for the staff. Forty per cent of all the paediatric nurses who train in Britain come from the Charles West School of Nursing. The importance of the nursing staff is recognised more than ever. Love and devotion to children are still needed, but are not now sufficient in themselves. Looking after children in

however, Great Ormond Street was always more relaxed in its attitude to parents than most hospitals, many of which, even in the 1950s, banned visitors to children. Certainly children's hospitals are now much more friendly places and a stay in hospital is less of an ordeal for the child, however worrying it is for parents.

It is doubtful whether children can always understand why they are in hospital, especially since often complicated technology is used in their treatment. A conversation between two children overheard in Great Ormond Street illustrates this:

First child: 'Are you a medical or a surgical patient?'
Second child: 'Sorry, but I don't really understand.'
First child: 'I mean were you ill when you came here or did they make you ill afterwards?'

The growing number of women doctors at Great Ormond Street and elsewhere may have contributed towards this humanising effect. Great Ormond Street approaches the emotional and traumatic problems of child and parents with sympathy, help and impressive success, despite the fact that patients are usually sent on from other hospitals and need the most advanced diagnosis and treatment for exceedingly rare illnesses and abnormalities.

The Wishing Well Appeal

The hospital wanted to develop in several areas. There was a need to accommodate mothers more easily and comfortably instead of in makeshift beds and places, to provide total family care, and have more space in ward cubicles for up-to-date equipment and monitoring instruments. So the Wishing Well Appeal for the redevelopment of Great Ormond Street was launched in 1987.

Great advances had been made in paediatric and neonatal surgery enabling congenital heart defects and other mal-

intensive care demands high standards of training and skill. Much of Great Ormond Street's success in completely involving parents in their children's treatment is due to the expertise and understanding of the nursing staff.

At Queen Elizabeth Hospital an academic unit set up in 1972 teaches undergraduate students from the medical colleges of St Bartholomew's and the London Hospitals, and is also linked with the Institute of Child Health; in the same year the Queen opened the Hayward Building for diagnostic investigations and research; and more recently the Donald Winnicott Centre for physically and mentally handicapped children also opened adjacent to Queen Elizabeth Hospital.

Earlier, in 1969, the Wolfson Centre, also for counselling and treating handicapped children and their families, had been opened as a branch of the Institute on a part of the old Foundling Hospital site in Coram's Fields. The fact that it was next to such a famous children's playground was symbolic of Charles West's belief in the importance of play in the recovery of sick children. Great Ormond Street has always recognised this, with play leaders and play areas for

101 The Square, St Bartholomew's Hospital, West Smithfield, London, in 1844.

every ward and department, and a large playroom and an open-air playground. After forty years part of the dream of 1929 had come true in a very small way.

But an earlier and fully realised dream came to an end in 1984, when Tadworth Court separated. More and more of the hospital's restricted revenue was being spent on comparatively few patients in Surrey. Similar problems nearly fifty years earlier had threatened the closure of Tadworth Court in 1938. As the children there were nearly all acute or long-stay orthopaedic and other cases, it was a heart-breaking decision for many members of the board and staff. In 1984 the hospital transferred all the buildings and equipment and over a quarter of the extensive grounds to the newly formed Tadworth Court Trust. Queen Mary's Hospital for Children in Carshalton took over the treatment of the orthopaedic patients, which solved one important problem. Under its own separate charity and management, Tadworth Court became, in fact, more fully used. It still continues one important function in providing periods of relief for the families of badly handicapped or retarded children by looking after the child for a while. A number of Great Ormond Street's doctors still gave their services to Tadworth even after it had become separated.

The children's response

At Great Ormond Street the wards, operating theatres and many other departments could no longer be altered and adapted to modern paediatric demands and technology. Even after the Government had made a substantial contribution of around £25 million, it was estimated that the Wishing Well Appeal for the hospital's reconstruction would need to raise £30 million. The chances of achieving this seemed remote, especially when the sum was later raised to £42 million. What happened was one of the most wonderful things in the history of Great Ormond Street. Under the joint patronage of the Prince and Princess of Wales, an enormously sympathetic response to Great Ormond Street's need came from every corner of the country and from overseas. Charles West's remark about Dickens, like a good fairy, having given the hospital the gift of winning love and favour everywhere was prophetic for our time. The appeal was named after the fountain which had stood in the old hospital garden, into which the children would throw their few coppers and wish to get better and be able to play again with all

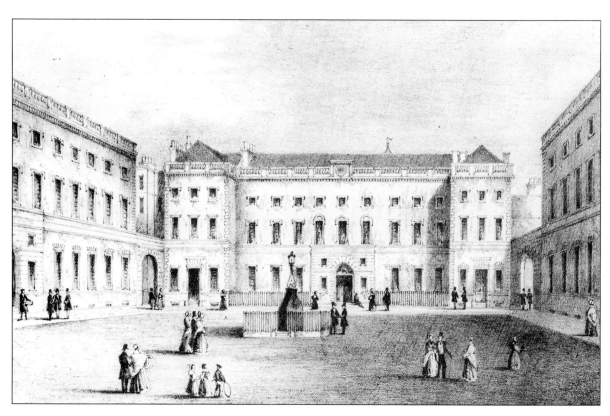

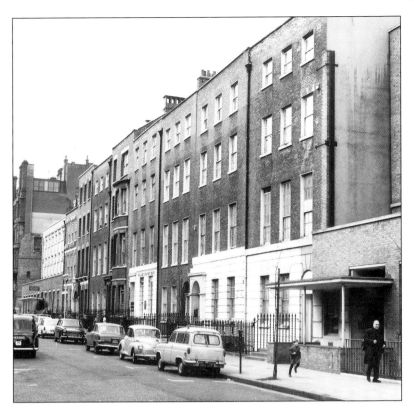

102 The north side of Great Ormond Street in 1967. The Charles West School of Nursing moved into a new building in 1960 (far right). The old houses between the school and the out-patients department accommodated various departments of the hospital and also served as a nurses' home. Williams Deacon's Bank (centre) has been the hospital's bank since its inception (now The Royal Bank of Scotland). This side of the street was rebuilt soon after this photograph was taken.

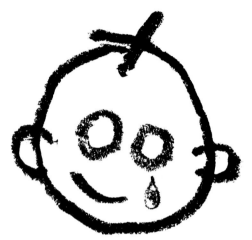

103 The Wishing Well Appeal logo.

their little friends. This fountain, as Dr Poynton remembered, was known and loved all over the world, and its modern symbolical resurrection produced a similarly warm response. An unusually high proportion of the money raised came in small donations. But the most touching response of all, which made everyone connected with the appeal feel both humble and proud, was the overwhelming support from children, who everywhere adopted Great Ormond Street as their own. They gave sums ranging from a few pennies of precious pocket money to thousands of pounds raised by ingenious and almost incredible schemes of sponsorship, or collected with unflagging enthusiasm by schools.

By a curious coincidence the BBC television programme about the appeal, *A Fighting Chance*, which did so much to publicise it, was broadcast on the last day of 1987, when the copyright of *Peter Pan* officially expired in Great Britain and most other countries. On 10 March 1988 the House of Lords moved an amendment to a new copyright bill then passing through Parliament. This gave Great Ormond Street the right to receive royalties from *Peter Pan* for ever. It was a unique and marvellous privilege, something that no other book or play has ever or will ever be granted, and certainly no other hospital. But then there is only one

Peter Pan and only one Great Ormond Street.

The Wishing Well Appeal reached its target nearly a year ahead of schedule. It was the most successful appeal ever known, not only in the hospital's history, but in the whole history of fundraising. The wealth of sympathy it revealed for children in hospital will, it is hoped, benefit all children everywhere. A Peter Pan Children's Fund has been launched to raise funds not only for Great Ormond Street, but also for other children's hospitals and paediatric research in Britain and in North America, and eventually in other parts of the world. It will make *Peter Pan*'s opening words 'All children except one grow up', come true not only in the Never-Never-Land of story, but in the grim world of deprivation and disease which is often so near.

TIME CHART

AD
1922 Great Ormond Street starts research department for children's diseases.
1942 Beveridge Report published. Great Ormond Street plans Institute of Child Health.
1945 Dr Alan Moncrieff becomes first professor of child health.
1946 Institute of Child Health begins work at Great Ormond Street. Hospital School at Tadworth.
1948 National Health Service begins. World Health Organization founded.
1951 Hospital school at Great Ormond Street.
1952 HM The Queen visits Great Ormond Street for its centenary. Great Ormond Street encourages mothers to visit children frequently.
1953 Great Ormond Street starts sending doctors and nurses to Africa, Middle East, etc.
1954 New out-patient department opened.
1959 Platt Report recommends unrestricted visiting by parents.
1960 Charles West School of Nursing moves into new building.
1962 Great Ormond Street frontage to Out-patient Department developed.

1964 Barrie Wing opened.
1965 Institute of Child Health moves to own building in Guilford Street.
1968 Queen Elizabeth Hospital for Children joined with Great Ormond Street.
1969 Wolfson Centre opened next to Coram's Fields.
1972 Academic unit set up at Queen Elizabeth Hospital. Hayward Building opened.
1978 Donald Winnicott Centre opened.
1982 Special health authorities formed for postgraduate hospitals.
1984 Tadworth Court separates and becomes a special trust.
1987 Wishing Well Appeal started under joint patronage of Prince and Princess of Wales.
1988 Great Ormond Street granted continued right to royalties from *Peter Pan*. Cardiac Wing opened.
1989 Wishing Well Appeal reaches its target of £42 million a year ahead of schedule.
1991 Princess of Wales lays foundation stone of new clinical building.

CHAPTER 9

Reaching for the Stars

One of the diseases which defied both penicillin and the sulphonamide drugs was tuberculosis. Despite progress made in its control since Koch discovered the tubercle bacillus in 1882 and finally demonstrated its infectious nature, tuberculosis was still in the 1930s a principal cause of mortality in children between 5 and 15 years of age. After Koch's discovery, Great Ormond Street, like other hospitals, took extra precautions and much later a special tuberculosis ward was opened. Notification of tuberculosis to local medical officers of health became compulsory in 1911 for England and Wales. At the same time, the Astor Committee launched a comprehensive national tuberculosis service of clinics, dispensaries, hospital beds and sanatoria. This, together with improved housing and X-ray screening in communities and schools, slowed the spread of infection. In 1908 William Waldorf Astor had given Great Ormond Street a new out-patients department in memory of his little daughter, who had died from tuberculosis. Now, with the new service to hospitals, the Astor family's concern was being demonstrated at national level.

From 1900, surgery to collapse and rest the infected lung was an option, but many thought it unsuitable for children. At the Pasteur Institute, Calmette and Guérin developed the BCG vaccine and began injecting children in 1924. Although it is now an accepted precaution, its use was controversial for many years. Infected milk was a common cause of non-pulmonary tuberculosis in children's glands and bones. Tests and inspections on all dairy cows began in the 1930s, and tubercle-free herds were slowly established. These and the pasteurisation of nearly all milk led to the virtual eradication of bovine tuberculosis. But although these measures reduced the incidence of tuberculosis, it was still a serious problem. Between 1939 and 1941, under wartime conditions, deaths from tuberculosis in Great Britain increased by eighteen per cent to 32,841. These included 2,871 children.

Streptomycin – a valuable discovery

The discovery of penicillin started an intensive search for other antibiotics. S. A. Waksman of Rutgens University, New Brunswick, a soil microbiologist, headed a team, including A. Schatz and Elizabeth Bugie, that set out to find an antibiotic effective against tuberculosis. They tested many thousands of soil cultures before discovering streptomycin in 1943. Towards the end of their investigation, a daughter of one of the research team was stricken with tuberculous meningitis, then very often fatal. The girl was treated with streptomycin for four months and became the first human to be cured of tuberculous meningitis by an antibiotic.

In 1947 Great Ormond Street was one of eight hospitals taking part in a trial of streptomycin on acute miliary tuberculosis, a dangerous form with infection that spread rapidly. It proved of great value. Used against tuberculous meningitis, a success rate of over fifty per cent was achieved, a vast improvement on any previous method. When doctors at Great Ormond Street saw a lethargic and suffering child, formerly with little hope of recovery, become alert and happier, and younger children beginning to walk around their cots after only a month of treatment, they could understand something Waksman was to say later.

After receiving the Nobel prize in 1952, Waksman visited many European hospitals. In the grounds of the Hôpital Sâlpetrière in Paris, he was photographed accepting flowers from two little children who had been saved by his streptomycin. 'As I patted their lovely curly heads I felt like crying,' Waksman remembered. 'I looked back to see the two little ones waving goodbye. This was enough compensation for all the sleepless nights and endless days spent in the study of the lowly microbes of the soil.'

An aid to recovery

Doctors at Great Ormond Street soon realised that the long months (at least three and sometimes nine) of often painful injections necessary for a cure imposed a great strain on the child. 'Frequent and regular visits by parents are called for once improvement has started, and every device used for keeping the child happy and contented.' This was an early recognition that unrestricted visiting by parents played an important role in a child's recovery.

It was noticed that the tubercle bacilli could develop a strong resistance to streptomycin, especially over extended periods of treatment. Sometimes giddiness and deafness were a side-effect. Other antibiotics were developed, such as isoniazid, which in combination with streptomycin overcame most of the disadvantages, and produced even better results. Waksman's discovery completely changed the treatment of tuberculosis. In 1954 it was found that deaths from tuberculosis in Great Britain had fallen by sixty-five per cent in five years.

Since the discoveries of Fleming and Waksman many other antibiotics have been found which have helped to destroy or inhibit nearly all the infections caused by bacteria and fungi. Countless drugs have been discovered and synthesized to combat other diseases, malfunctions, deficiencies and nervous disorders. Without drugs to overcome the body's natural rejection of alien organs and tissue, transplants would not be possible. Recently drugs have been developed to work the other way, by helping patients whose own immune systems are malfunctioning because of AIDS or cancer.

Against cancer, the first cytotoxic drugs were developed which inhibited the growth of malignant cells, and chemotherapy became an alternative and a reinforcement to treatment by radiotherapy. Unfortunately, the cytotoxic drugs only worked at the cost of harming some of the body's own cells. Children undergoing chemotherapy for leukaemia could, for instance, have their kidneys damaged. Nausea and hair-loss are more common though minor consequences. Research has found improved anti-cancer drugs. Among the latest are the platinum anti-cancer drugs and carboplatin, which is less toxic in its side-effects. These and others are being tested.

Work on viruses

A large volume would be needed to list all the new drugs which have been found, researched and developed in the last thirty years or so. Despite some tragic mistakes, such as the sedative thalidomide which resulted in thousands of children being born with severely shortened arms and legs, the immense advances in medicine and surgery over the last forty years would not have been possible without many of these new drugs. Virus-caused diseases, however, seem to be unaffected by any antibiotic or chemical drug; vaccination, originated by Edward Jenner over a century and a half ago, remains the only method of control. Recent research into the nucleic acids has made it possible to introduce synthetic strains of DNA into bacteria to produce specific proteins, including interferon. As interferon is released from the virus-infected cell into the bloodstream, it can enter an uninfected cell and stop the virus entering and multiplying itself in turn. So it plays a large part in the body's immunity against viral diseases. Interferon can now be used against some lymphomas (one of the most common cancers in the young) and solid tumours. Further research, in which the Institute of Child Health has participated, may help in new measures against viruses.

Work on viruses received a fresh impetus when John Enders, Frederick

104 In the 1920s splints for encasing the limbs of patients suffering from poliomyelitis were made in the hospital in the 'non-inflammable splint shop'.

Robbins and Thomas Wheeler, working at the Boston Children's Hospital, managed to cultivate the poliomyelitis virus, one of the smallest known, in test-tubes, outside an animal host, in 1949. Four years later Dr Jonas Salk had prepared a vaccine of the dead poliomyelitis virus, which gave protection and immunity when tested in his laboratory. His own three children were the first to be vaccinated against infantile paralysis, as poliomyelitis was called. Within another four years many millions of children all over the world had been successfully immunised. Meanwhile Dr Albert Sabin had developed a safe form of live attenuated vaccine which could be given orally to children on sugar lumps or in sweets. The success of these two vaccines can be measured by the fact that in 1957 England and Wales had nearly 5,000 cases of poliomyelitis, but by 1967 there were under 30. In 1968, Great Ormond Street had seen only three cases in eight years, all in unvaccinated children.

The treatment of poliomyelitis

Infantile paralysis was a viral infection which mostly attacked children, sometimes leading to a permanent paralysis of muscles and limbs. It had been known for centuries. It was illustrated on an

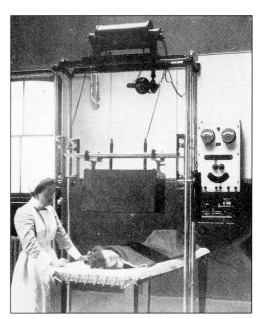

105 A patient receiving 'electrical treatment' for infantile paralysis (poliomyelitis) in 1911.

ancient Egyptian relief. Michael Underwood first described it in 1789. Charles West gave an early accurate account of it as 'morning paralysis'. There was no real remedy for the lamed children, although fresh air and an encouragement of movement was sometimes recommended. Great Ormond Street saw many children who had been lamed by poliomyelitis. Before 1914, the hospital's Dr Batten devised a form of lightweight splint made from a specially strong non-inflammable form of celluloid called Pexuloid, which was invented by the

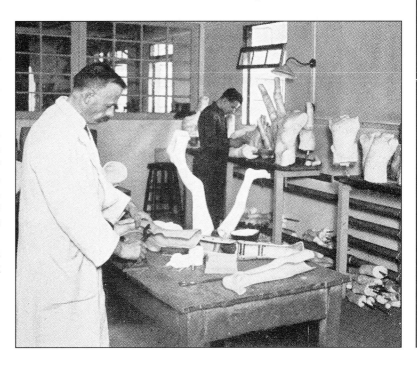

hospital's indefatigable and omniscient head pharmacist, Wicliffe Peck. These splints encouraged the child to walk at an early stage after illness. Poliomyelitis in modern times seemed to attack the more prosperous communities, who had not acquired immunity in infancy. A famous example was Franklin D. Roosevelt, the American president: at 39 he was attacked by the disease and became paralysed from the waist down.

If the disease attacked the respiratory muscles the victim was unable to breathe. Although various attempts had been made earlier at artificial respiration, mostly for victims of drowning, it was Dr Woillez, a physician in Northern France, who first devised the idea of the patient's body being entirely enclosed in a steel cylinder, his head protruding, with a rubber collar round the neck for an airtight seal. A hand-operated pump worked the 'spirophore', as Dr Woillez named it, the true forerunner of the iron lung, raising and lowering the pressure in the cylinder. It was first demonstrated in 1876, and used in some cases of drowning, though with little success. Over the next fifty years various other methods and types of apparatus were devised, but none proved really practical.

106 A respirator, or 'iron lung', in use at the hospital during the 1930s.

The first iron lung

The idea of making a reliable breathing machine for use in respiratory failure caused by poliomyelitis gained more attention in the 1920s. It was in 1928, obviously directly inspired by Woillez's spirophore, that Professor Philipp Drinker and I. A. Shaw invented at Harvard the first satisfactory version of the iron lung. This became known as the Drinker Respirator. Drinker Respirators were used over the next few years to treat over a hundred cases of poliomyelitis in Boston. In New York, during the same period, twenty machines treated not only poliomyelitis cases, more than at Boston, but also scores of respiratory failure from other causes, such as gas poisoning and electric shock. In both cities the Drinker Respirator had proved itself.

Professor Drinker brought one of his machines to England in May 1931, placing it in the London School of Hygiene, where it was demonstrated and made available for use. It was called for and operated several times, offering relief but not ultimate success. Late one night in 1932 it was rushed down to Oxford, where it was used on a boy from Stowe School with respiratory paralysis from poliomyelitis. His was the first life saved

in this country by the Drinker Respirator. A little later it was called for by the National Hospital, Queen Square, where again a child's life was saved. It was still the only machine in the country. In 1933 ICI sponsored certain modifications to the machine and presented one to Great Ormond Street, and shortly afterwards gave a second machine to a general hospital.

At Great Ormond Street two small children with infantile paralysis and respiratory complications were soon successfully treated by the Drinker Respirator. It was put to good use in succeeding years, especially during the poliomyelitis epidemic of 1938. In that year, Both, an Australian engineer, built a more economical form of cabinet respirator. It was made from laminated wood, and was easier to handle. Lord Nuffield, whose contributions to medical charity and research were numerous and legendary (he contributed £50,000 towards the cost of the new Great Ormond Street building which opened that year) immediately became interested. Seven hundred of these Both respirators were built in the Nuffield car works, and donated to various hospitals throughout Britain and the Commonwealth – a very practical example of philanthropy. After the war, in 1947, several respirators were in use at Great Ormond Street. In Sweden, during the poliomyelitis epidemic of 1951, Professor Lassen and Dr Ibsen thought of applying the latest anaesthetic techniques, used to respire patients when curare was administered, to a respiratory machine. From this came the prototype of the modern ventilator. All this was important in the development of intensive care. Two or three years later, in 1954, the first successful transfer of a kidney from a living donor was made between identical adult twins by Dr Joseph Murray at Boston.

Intensive care

The first intensive coronary care units were started in Britain by Professor Shillingford in the early 1960s. Around the same time intensive care was being carried out at Great Ormond Street in its congenital heart unit, by Dr Bonham Carter and his colleagues. (Professor Christiaan Barnard performed the world's

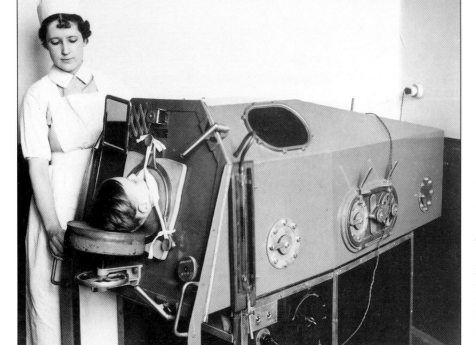

first successful heart transplant operation at Cape Town in 1967.) Great Ormond Street's first intensive care unit as such was opened in the Respiratory Ward by Dr A. P. Norman and Dr E. N. Hey during 1975.

The advance in scientific technology after 1945 had made such progress possible. The discovery of the transistor, the solid-state integrated circuit, and the use of silicon chips in microprocessors, for example, completely revolutionised electronics and computers. Unwieldy equipment, liable to frequent mechanical failure, was no longer needed for complex and continual medical monitoring, and much more sophisticated and detailed information could be recorded. Radiography also benefited from the changes, and was able to enlarge both its fields, diagnosis and therapy. With the help of radioisotope tracers radiologists can now pinpoint specific organs and cells, and follow the exact molecular processes of the living body. Body scanners incorporated computers, and were improved to use both ultrasound and magnetic resonance, giving in effect three-dimensional images of the brain, heart and other organs. Doctors could monitor the development of the unborn child within the mother's body, diagnosing possible defects and hereditary disorders.

Lasers used in diagnosis

As well as improved X-rays, there was the power of lasers available; these could be used not only as a surgical tool, but also as a help in diagnosis. Laser scanners are now being made which show details which cannot be distinguished by even the most powerful electron-microscope. Cardiac catheterisation, which had begun experimentally before 1939, became a routine procedure, using modern materials and discoveries, such as fibre optics; the principle was extended to improved endoscopes, oesophagoscopes and bronchoscopes for examining and viewing the interior of body cavities, and the stomach and the lungs, without the need for surgery. Non-intrusive investigation is being increasingly used, and non-intrusive surgery with the help of lasers,

ultrasound, and the advance of nano-technology (micromachinery computers and sensors on the minutest possible scale) has become practical.

The artificial kidney machine (which used the process of dialysis discovered by Thomas Graham a century before) kept alive patients with chronic kidney failure. At Great Ormond Street, for instance, seventy-six children with acute renal failure were treated by dialysis during 1988. Kidney machines and heart–lung machines, greatly extended the range of surgery. Open-heart surgery became almost commonplace, and with the help of microsurgical techniques organ transplants were carried out at various hospitals with increasing success. Artificial materials and plastics had already enabled the surgeon to repair defective and worn-out sections of the blood-vessels, to give people artificial joints, and to insert pace-makers to regulate heartbeats.

Neonatal and paediatric surgery went from strength to strength at Great Ormond Street. The Spitz-Holter valve operation for relieving excess brain fluid in hydrocephalus and spina bifida, first done at the Philadelphia Children's Hospital in 1955, was introduced into England by George Macnab. Another important breakthrough was the operation for oesophageal atresia, a congenital restriction or obstruction of the gullet, which D. J. Waterston perfected at the hospital in the 1960s. By 1968 over one thousand infants had been operated on for congenital heart diseases. Open-heart surgery, possible because of improved intensive care, was increasingly undertaken. During 1971 at Great Ormond Street, 222 open-heart operations were performed, 55 of them on infants under 12 months old, with 80 per cent success. In that year a new heart–lung machine was being built to the hospital's own design, which met the special needs of babies and children, and Professor Christiaan Barnard, the pioneer of heart transplants, was one of many distinguished visitors to the hospital. But the main emphasis was still to be on complex congenital heart malformations, such as blue babies, hole-in-the-heart children and new-born infants with their two great arteries transposed. In March 1988, collaborating with Papworth Hospital, Great Ormond Street began a heart–lung transplant programme; and in that year kidney transplants, some on

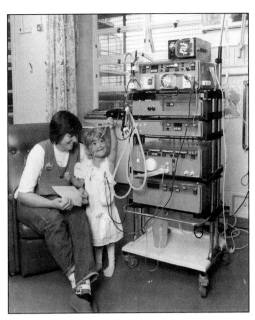

107 A young patient with play specialist Lesley and a kidney dialysis machine.

children under 5 years of age, were successfully made.

Apart from cardiac and neurosurgical disorders and anomalies which are dealt with in their own special units, the neonatal surgical unit at Great Ormond Street, much the largest such unit in the country, treats over 220 new-born infants every year for a wide range of congenital abnormalities.

Cystic fibrosis – treatment and research

One hereditary disease with which the hospital has been concerned for many years is cystic fibrosis. In this disease, the affected cells cannot get rid of chloride and other natural salts, and so a thick mucus is produced. This obstructs the pancreas and the intestinal glands, and malnutrition results because the production of digestive enzymes is hindered. The mucus also blocks the bronchial tubes, making chest infections a constant problem. Previously it was often fatal, but today with treatment including antibiotics and pancreatic enzymes, daily physiotherapy and a controlled diet, most children now reach adulthood. Together with Queen Elizabeth Hospital for Children, Great Ormond Street is the regional centre for such treatment, and Tadworth Court still cares for in-patients with cystic fibrosis,

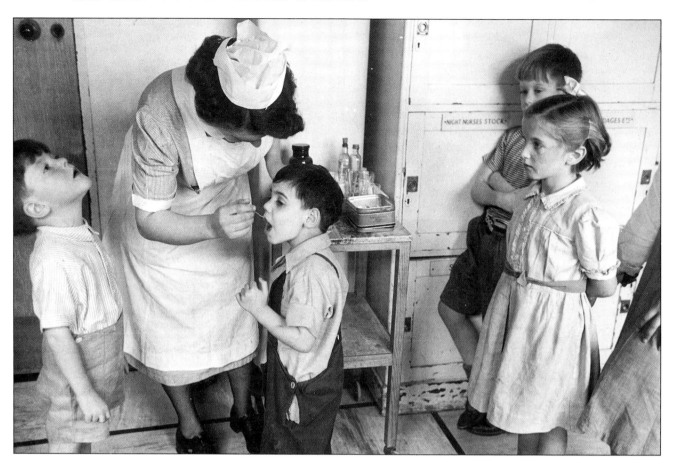

108 Open wide! Medicine time on one of the wards in 1952.

INBORN ERRORS OF METABOLISM

The Croonian Lectures delivered before the Royal College of Physicians of London, in June, 1908

By
ARCHIBALD E. GARROD
D.M., M.A. OXON.

Fellow of the Royal College of Physicians,
Assistant Physician to, and Lecturer on Chemical Pathology
at St. Bartholomew's Hospital,
Physician to the Hospital for Sick Children,
Great Ormond Street

" ἐν πᾶσι τοῖς φυσικοῖς ἔνεστί τι θαυμαστόν."
Aristotle, Περὶ ζῴων μορίων, I. 5.

LONDON
HENRY FROWDE   HODDER & STOUGHTON
OXFORD UNIVERSITY PRESS   20, WARWICK SQUARE, E.C.
1909

109 Dr (later Sir) Archibald Garrod's discoveries revolutionised ideas concerning genetics.

as it did before the separation from Great Ormond Street. Gene diagnosis before birth and, in North America, experimental gene therapy, are being researched. Heart–lung transplants for cystic fibrosis are now successfully carried out where appropriate at Great Ormond Street.

Children with cancer can now be much more reasonably assured of a cure, but careful monitoring is needed to catch and minimise any possible later complications from the effects of treatment. The first real success in bone marrow transplants at the hospital was in 1968. Today over three-quarters of these patients prosper. Since 1983 it has been possible even before the baby is born to detect the deficiency in immunity that will make such transplants necessary. Great Ormond Street was the first hospital to do this, but this and other medical advances are not really due to one doctor, one scientist or even one hospital. Medical research has grown from the individual genius of the nineteenth century, through research teams based on a single laboratory or institution, to the present world-wide investigations and exchange of information, which can now be passed on at the speed of light.

Much remains to be done, because medical research is never-ending. Although between eighty and ninety per cent of the children in intensive care now survive, of those that die, nearly half do so in the first forty-eight hours. This has become a major research area at Great Ormond Street, as is another field: the investigation of children with HIV infections (AIDS).

Space technology and medicine

Exactly a generation ago, on 12 April 1961, Yuri Gagarin was the first human to pass through the hitherto inexorable barrier between earth and space. Medicine is also reaching for the stars. The same science and technology that helped flight into space has helped medicine to master the infinitely little in the development of molecular biology, the most important step forward of all. Sir Peter Medawar has said: 'Nothing has occurred to shake my belief that the discovery of the structure and functions of the nucleic acids is the greatest achievement of science in the twentieth century.'

The nucleic acids are DNA and RNA which store genetic information in all living organisms, and make up the double helix of the genetic code. This code is the same for the countless millions of living things, from the simplest and most minute of organisms to the complex structure of animals and humans. It unlocks the ultimate mystery of life.

New horizons in medicine

Research on the nucleic acids has revolutionised medical genetics and medicine itself. Molecular biology and genetic engineering saw unlimited horizons unfolding. Already we have seen the practical results of investigations into fields once thought unapproachable. That revolution began with Sir Archibald Garrod, who was a physician at Great Ormond Street and assistant physician at St Bartholomew's in 1908, the year he gave a series of lectures at the Royal College of Physicians. Under the title *Inborn Errors of Metabolism* he set out

what became a fundamental concept in medical genetics, that of congenital deficiencies of enzymes due to particular genes or hereditary factors. This is, of course, an over-simplification of a very complex subject, and to follow its development through to the present day is far beyond the scope of this book.

Garrod was ahead of his time. He was rather like Einstein, who three years before, in 1905, had published four papers, including his special theory of relativity, which were so revolutionary in their concept that their importance was not really appreciated until some years later. Garrod's work also had to wait for recognition. He was, however, appointed regius professor of medicine at Oxford in 1920, succeeding the great Sir William Osler. Both Einstein and Max Planck (the originator of quantum theory in 1900) needed the development of scientific techniques to confirm their revolutionary approach to physics. When this happened the world and the cosmos were never the same again. Garrod, whose work belongs to almost the same period as these two mathematical geniuses, had to wait somewhat longer until the advance of molecular biology, and then medicine was never the same again. He had been dead for twenty-two

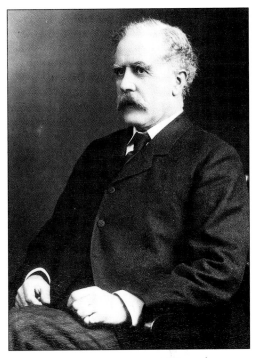

110 Sir Archibald Garrod (1857–1936).

years when G. W. Beadle shared with E. L. Tatum and J. Lederberg a 1958 Nobel Prize. This was awarded for their work on the way in which the chromosomes in the cell nucleus transmit inherited characters. Beadle wrote: 'In this long roundabout way we had rediscovered what Garrod had seen so clearly so many years before.'

Today nearly half the children referred to Great Ormond Street, often after being seen by many doctors and other hospitals, are ill because of genetic disorders, some very rare. The hospital and the Institute of Child Health have long specialised in this area, and it is recognised that usually in these cases only they can help the desperately ill child and its increasingly worried parents.

In the first chapter it was said that many of the great advances in medicine first involved and concerned children. The fact that Garrod, who joined Great Ormond Street almost exactly a century ago, also took charge, in 1904, of the children's department at St Bartholomew's is of great significance. 'No man is an island,' preached John Donne, poet and dean of St Paul's Cathedral, at a time when Galileo and William Harvey were leading science and medicine towards the modern world. Today, no sick child is an island, and each child's death concerns and affects us all.

TIME CHART

AD

1789 Michael Underwood first describes poliomyelitis.
1876 Dr Woillez devises the spirophor, the forerunner of the iron lung.
1882 Koch discovers tubercle bacillus.
1897 Notification of tuberculosis compulsory in New York and voluntary in Lancashire towns.
1900 Max Planck expounds quantum theory.
1905 Einstein publishes first paper on relativity.
1908 Archibald Garrod lectures, *Inborn Errors of Metabolism.*
1911 Notification of tuberculosis compulsory in England and Wales. National Health Insurance Act.
1924 Calmette and Guérin begin injecting children with BCG vaccine.
1926 Busch's work on magnetic coils makes electron microscope possible.
1928 The Drinker Respirator, first satisfactory iron lung.
1930 Inspection and tests on dairy cows begin.
1932 First life saved by a Drinker Respirator in England.
1933 Great Ormond Street given one of first Drinker Respirators. Irène Curie and F. Joliot produce radioactive isotopes.
1936–7 Work on electronic computer begins.
1938 Both cabinet respirator manufactured by Lord Nuffield. Borries and Ruska take first pictures of viruses with electron microscope.
1943 S. A. Waksman discovers streptomycin.
1947 Great Ormond Street takes part in a test of streptomycin.

1948 Transistors invented by Bardeen, Brattan and Shockley.
1949 John Enders cultivates poliomyelitis virus in test-tube.
1951 Lassen and Ibsen develop prototype of modern respirator.
1953–4 Jonas Salk produces vaccine against poliomyelitis.
1954 Joseph Murray makes first successful transplant of kidneys between identical twins. First use of radio-isotopes in medicine.
1958 Electronic computers introduced into research and commerce. G. W. Beadle shares Nobel Prize for work on chromosomes and genes.
1959 First bone-marrow bank started in Vienna.
1960s First intensive care coronary units started in Britain by Professor Shillingford. One started at Great Ormond Street in congenital heart unit.
1961 Yuri Gagarin first man in space.
1963 Vaccine against measles developed.
1967 Christiaan Barnard performs first successful heart transplant. Lasers used in surgery.
1970 Heart pace-makers first used.
1975 Respiratory intensive care unit opened at Great Ormond Street.
1983 Great Ormond Street detects immunity deficiencies in babies before birth.
1988 Great Ormond Street begins heart-lung transplant programme.
1991 Gene determining gender identified by British research team and female embryos of mice changed into males.

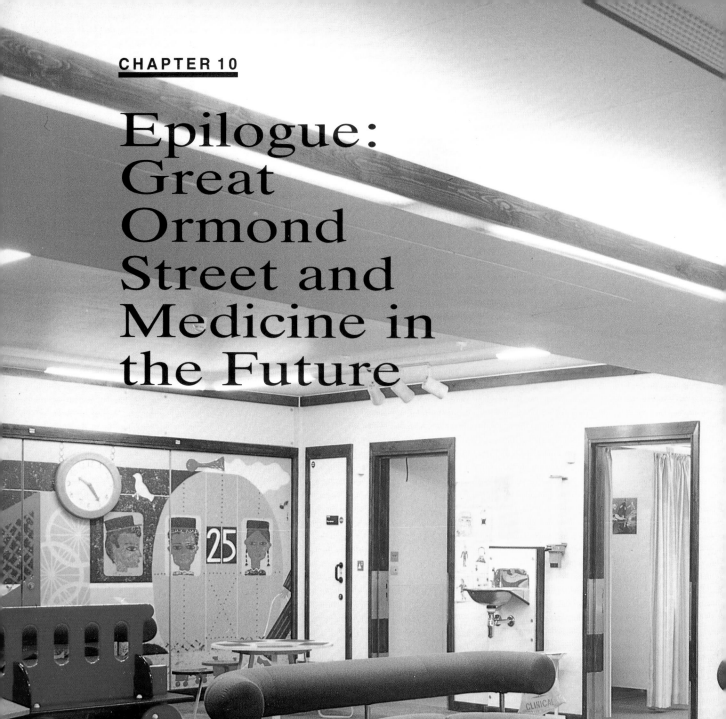

CHAPTER 10

Epilogue: Great Ormond Street and Medicine in the Future

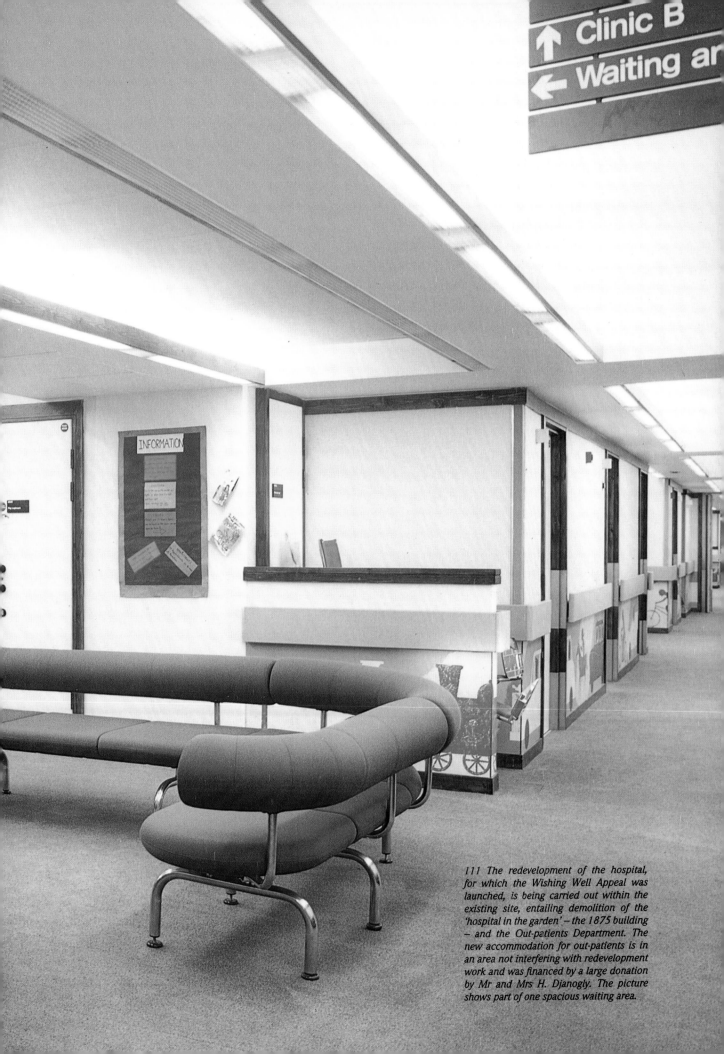

↑ Clinic B

← Waiting ar

INFORMATION

111 The redevelopment of the hospital, for which the Wishing Well Appeal was launched, is being carried out within the existing site, entailing demolition of the 'hospital in the garden' – the 1875 building – and the Out-patients Department. The new accommodation for out-patients is in an area not interfering with redevelopment work and was financed by a large donation by Mr and Mrs H. Djanogly. The picture shows part of one spacious waiting area.

What of the future? Medical research has gone far beyond the ability of any one individual or group to master. The mere mass of papers and reports covering every field and speciality, any one of which may contain information of vital importance to a worker in a hitherto unrelated area of research, needs the full resources of a globally interlinked computer-data system to become a help rather than a hindrance. Cybernetics, which is the study and analysis of information control and communication between all living things, especially man, machines and organisations, has already turned its attention to this and similar problems. The sifting, storage and cross-indexing of information is something modern computers can increasingly master. Already there are several international schemes and plans which intend to give computer access to all research information, apart from smaller and more limited information packs, such as MEDLINE, already in operation. It would seem that only questions of security can prevent the emergence of an actual 'HAL', the all-knowing, all-understanding, all-powerful computer solving every problem and controlling every action, as in the Arthur C. Clarke science fiction film *2001*. Perhaps its appearance will coincide with 2002, the 150th anniversary of the founding of the Hospital for Sick Children. At least that anniversary will mark a century and a half of medical progress without parallel. What a new century will bring stretches our imagination.

Into the twenty-first century

The hospital itself is being prepared for the twenty-first century. The new clinical building is already being built (see page 69), and soon a new laboratory block will follow. In recent years approximately 54,000 children have been treated every year as out-patients and over 12,500 a year as in-patients although the hospital is unable to use its full complement of 348 beds. When the reconstruction programme is complete, children at Great Ormond Street, both in-patients and out-patients, will have the benefit of a new and fully equipped modern hospital. It will be full of light from glazed passages overlooking courtyards, giving a sense of cheerfulness and space although all contained within the confines of the old site. The single-bed cubicles will have more room, not only for the necessary medical and monitoring equipment but also for a parent's bed to be permanently in place, instead of a temporary folding makeshift bed which is always in the way. All the wards, where possible, will have two playrooms, one for

112 The central courtyard of the new hospital will be light and airy.

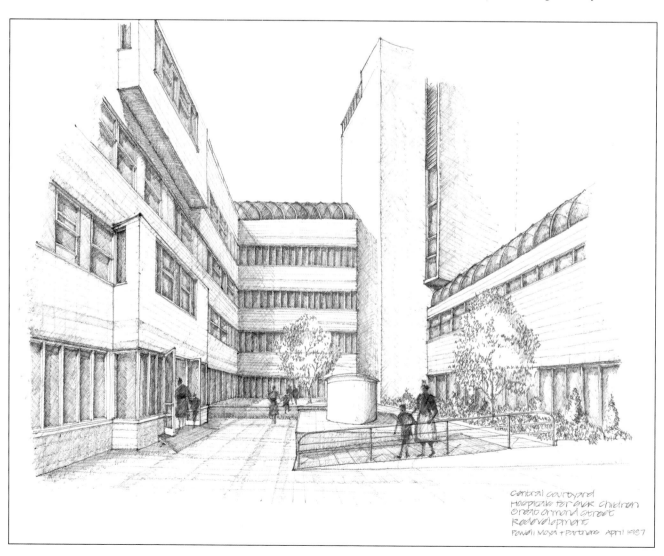

113 One feature of the new hospital will provide custom-built accommodation enabling a parent to stay with her or his child in hospital. This plan shows a typical single-bed ward with its own bathroom and bed for a parent.

THE HOSPITALS FOR SICK CHILDREN - GREAT ORMOND STREET

TYPICAL SINGLE BED WARD WITH AIRLOCK

INFECTIOUS DISEASES/IMMUNOLOGY

FLOOR PLAN

ELEVATION

Scale 1:20

toddlers and the other for teenagers, as these two age groups have vastly different needs. New operating theatres will be designed to complement and facilitate the use of the most advanced operating techniques and technology. There will be special transplant cubicles for children needing radical surgery and other treatment demanding absolutely sterile conditions with extensive precautions against any possibility of even the mildest infection.

The Hospitals for Sick Children and the Institute of Child Health will more than ever be combining their complementary functions – the most exacting clinical care and the most intensive research into children's diseases. It has been said that the clinical research of today is the clinical practice of tomorrow; but it is equally true that it is today's clinical practice which indicates and directs the research of tomorrow. Improvements in diagnostic procedure will certainly lead to greater emphasis on preventive medicine. The new chairs of international child health and of virology, both founded as part of the Wishing Well Appeal, will play a great part in this. Research into virus diseases, especially those of tropical origin, will increase.

Malaria – research continues

In the mid-1950s, the World Health Organization optimistically predicted that malaria would be wiped out within five years. Today, with the increasingly rapid development of resistance to even the latest anti-malarial drugs by the malaria parasite, the disease, once thought under control, is a serious and growing problem. Children make up most of the two million people estimated to die from malaria each year. This is but one field requiring urgent attention and new research. Genetically engineered vaccines, if all the ethical and technical problems can be overcome, may eventually do away with malaria, cancer,

heart disease, arthritis, mental illnesses and many other diseases which have stubbornly resisted the doctors and the scientists. Research trials are under way in hospitals and laboratories all over the world, but it is thought that effective and practical results will not come before the end of the century. Gene research may provide answers to sickle cell anaemia, Tay-Sach's disease, Alzheimer's disease and multiple sclerosis.

One consequence of research on nucleic acids is the development of biopharmaceuticals – drugs that can take the place of natural compounds in the body. They are specific in action and do not have side-effects. A technology that began in the 1970s, the first of these drugs to be produced by the chemical synthesis of proteins, or by cloning, included interferon, insulin and growth hormones. Other duplicates of natural

compounds to compensate for deficiencies will no doubt be found.

Surgery, using the extraordinary techniques which are becoming possible, will enlarge its scope, becoming increasingly non-intrusive or, to be more accurate, minimally invasive. Already angioplasty, where by using catheters a tiny balloon can be pumped up inside a narrowed blood-vessel to free the flow of blood, or even to repair a hole in the heart, has become an accepted procedure. At Great Ormond Street, neonatal and pre-natal surgery will occupy the forefront of research, together with investigations into the biology of surgical transplantation. Research into immunity deficiencies and HIV, together with the hospital's continuing emphasis on genetics and molecular medicine, will retain their importance, as will investigations into neurology and neuropsychology.

Text continued on page 70

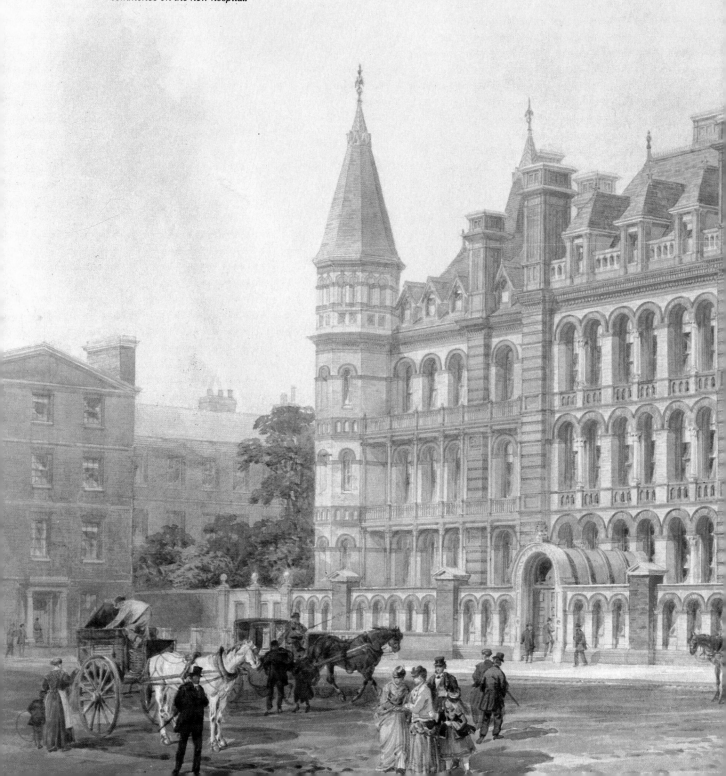

114 This building, designed by Edward M. Barry, was known as the 'hospital in the garden' because it was built in the gardens behind Nos. 48 and 49, Great Ormond Street, where the hospital was started. The side of one of the original houses can be seen on the right. The building was opened in 1875. It had many innovatory aspects including special facilities for the reception and treatment of infectious cases, nurses' accommodation and twin out-patient waiting halls. The far end of the building was demolished in 1936 to make room for the Southwood Building. The remainder was put to good use for another 54 years. It was demolished in 1990 to enable work to commence on the new hospital.

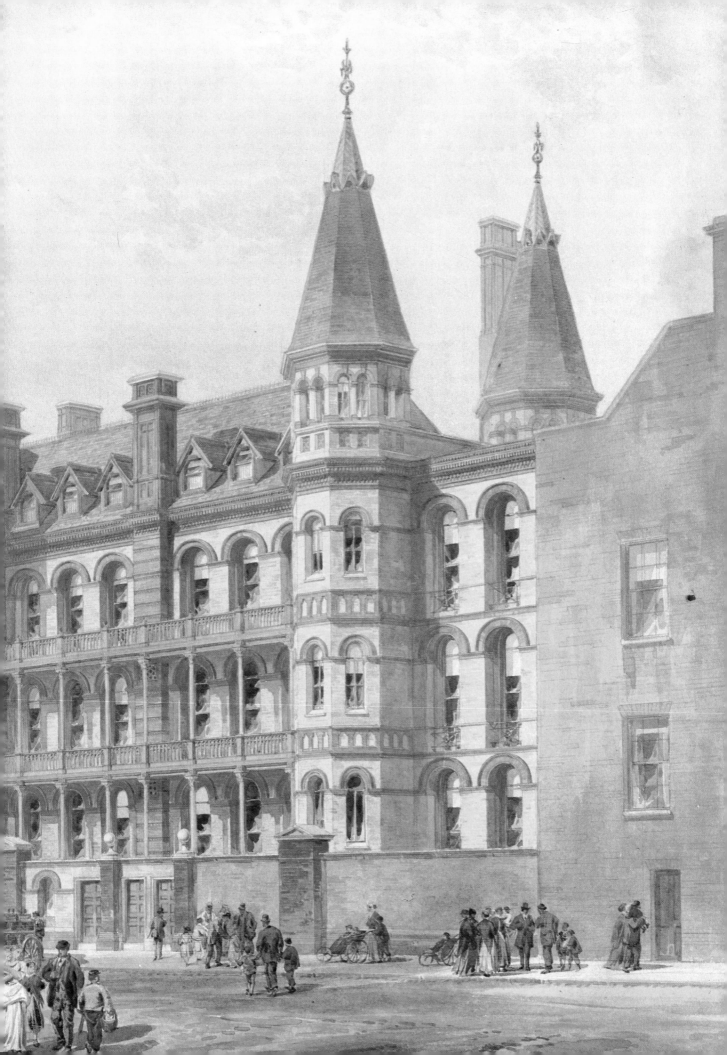

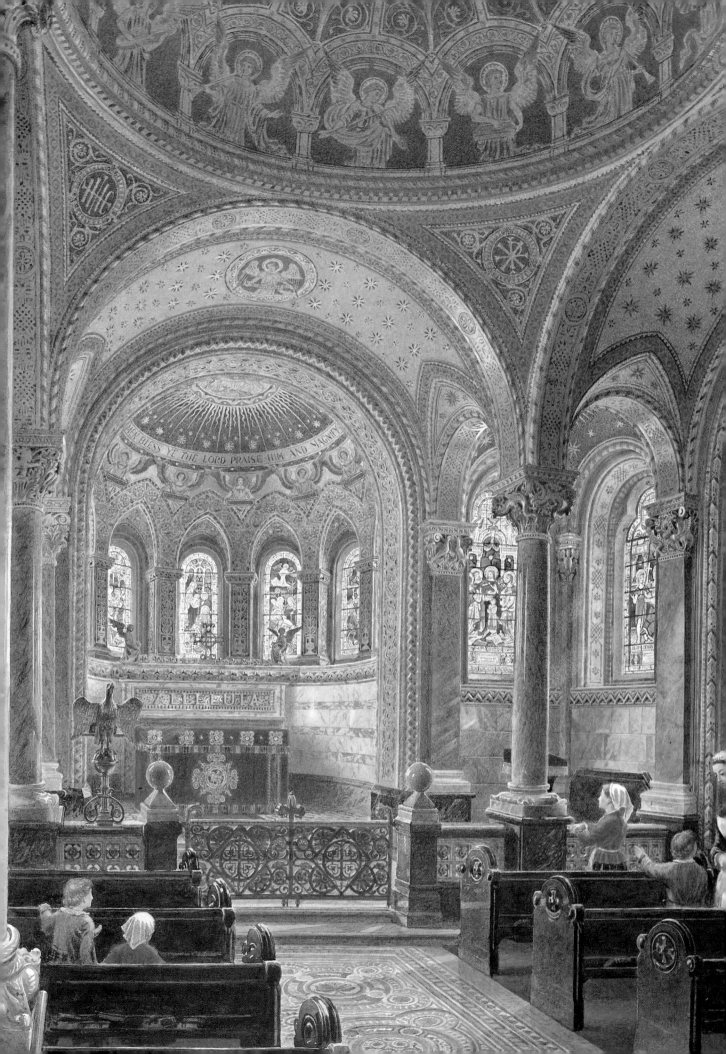

LEFT: *115 Chapel of St Christopher, the Hospital for Sick Children (watercolour by A. H. Haig, 1876). The first service held in the chapel was on the day before the official opening of the 'new' hospital on 18 November 1875. The chapel is designed in Byzantine style with ornately coloured and richly gilded frescoes and decorations on the walls and ceiling.*

RIGHT: *116 The Crimean War, 1854–56. An engraving showing Florence Nightingale in a ward at Scutari. The war started two years after the Hospital for Sick Children was opened and in the year that Charles West published his book about nursing sick children.*

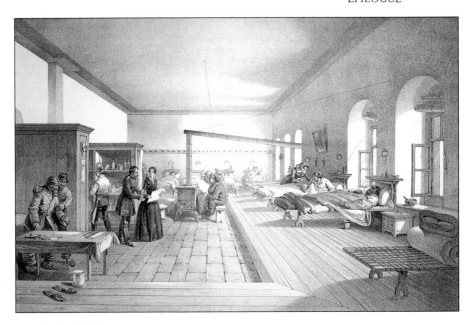

BELOW: 117 The Sick Room *by Mrs Emma Brownlow King. A painting of the Foundling Hospital contemporary with the early days of Great Ormond Street.*

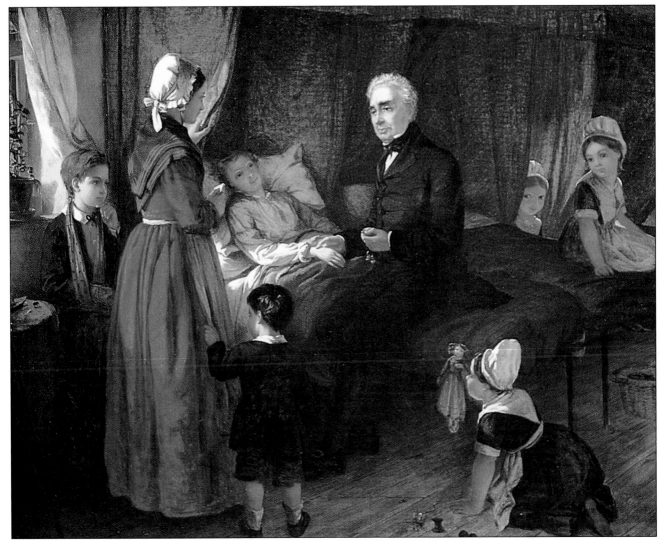

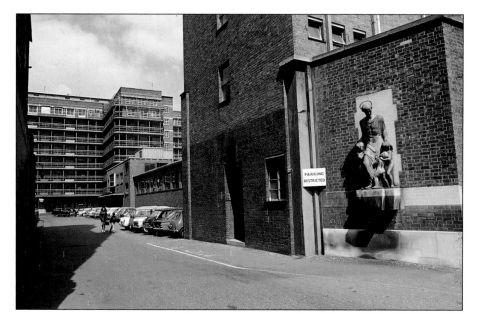

LEFT: *118 In 1954 the Out-patients Department was completed after sixteen years, the delay having been caused not only by the war but also by severe restrictions on building and building materials afterwards. From that time until 1989 this was the well-known and well-trodden hospital drive.*

BELOW: *119 By November 1990 the site was cleared and the Chapel of St Christopher moved to a new position.*

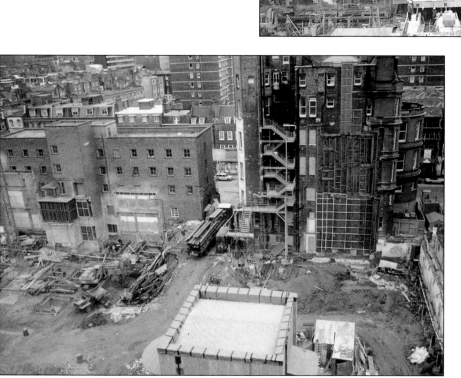

TOP RIGHT: *120 The new hospital under construction in Great Ormond Street (May 1991).*

BOTTOM RIGHT: *121 A model of the new hospital shows the South Wing building (1893) in the bottom left-hand corner, the Southwood Building (1937) at the top centre and the Cardiac Wing (1988) on the right-hand side. All the central area contains the new building fronting on to Powis Place.*

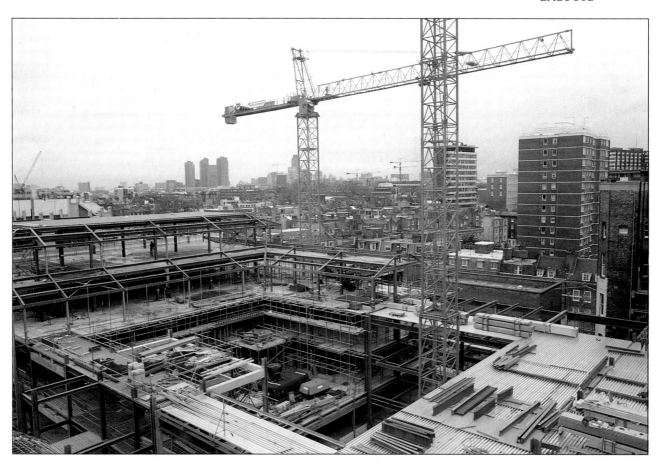

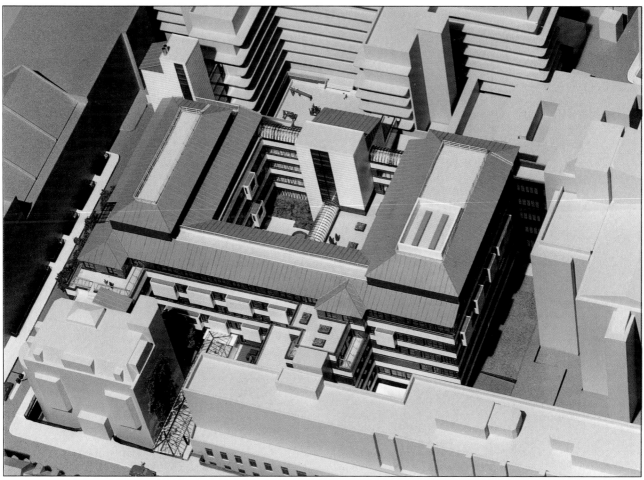

The child first and always

No one can really tell how medicine will develop. An unknown virus may suddenly cross the gap between humans and animals, as has happened in the immediate past, or even the gap between humans and plants. On the other hand, new and entirely different sciences and technologies may emerge from what were unrelated fields of research. The suggestions made above can only apply to the immediate future.

All would agree, however, that the hospital and the Institute will enlarge their joint participation in community medicine, offering advice, service and research on an international scale to help sick children in the Third World, as they already do in co-operation with the World Health Organization, UNICEF and other bodies. Work in Sri Lanka on cleft lip and cleft palate will form a model project on which to develop help for other abnormalities in other areas, not forgetting disease and deprivation of a more common kind.

It is the plight of the sick and famished child threatened by natural or man-made catastrophes which strikes hardest at the moral conscience of the world, cutting across all national boundaries, and ignoring the divisions of race, creed and politics. Could it be that the movement to help the sick child, which began in the children's dispensaries and children's hospitals at whose histories we have glanced, will in the world of the immediate future become the true message of hope and goodwill? Over the bed of the sick child, will we meet, bringing not only healing for the little ones, but also a remedy at last for all the folly and despair of a hitherto heedless and sick world?

122 This picture shows the complexity of the modern operating theatre in the Cardiac Wing of the hospital.

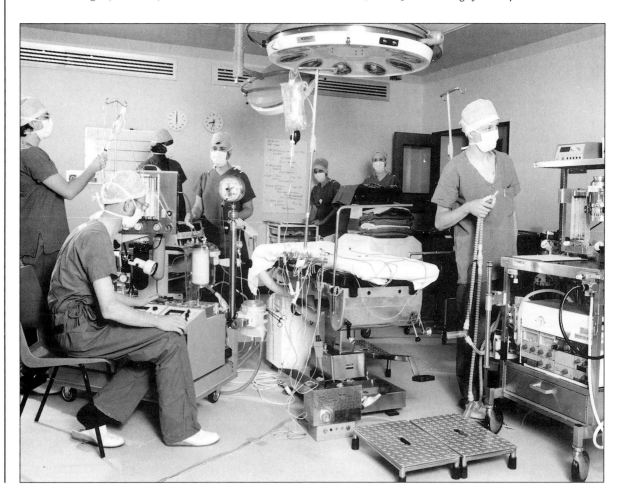

Index

Page numbers in bold type refer to illustrations and their captions

Start Science
Minibeasts

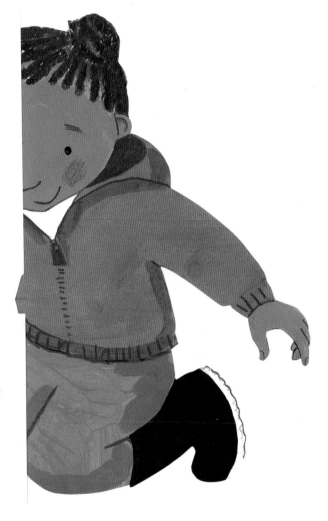

Sally Hewitt

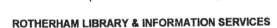

Chrysalis Children's Books

First published in the UK in 2003 by
Chrysalis Children's Books
An imprint of Chrysalis Books Group Plc
The Chrysalis Building, Bramley Road,
London W10 6SP

Paperback edition first published in 2005

ISBN 1 84138 270 1 (hb)
ISBN 1 84458 298 1 (pb)

British Library Cataloguing in Publication Data
for this book is available from the British Library.

Editorial manager: Joyce Bentley
Senior editor: Sarah Nunn
Project editor: Jean Coppendale
Designers: Rachel Hamdi, Holly Mann
Illustrators: Gwyneth Williamson, Joanna Partis
Educational consultants: Sally Morgan and
Helen Walters

Printed in China

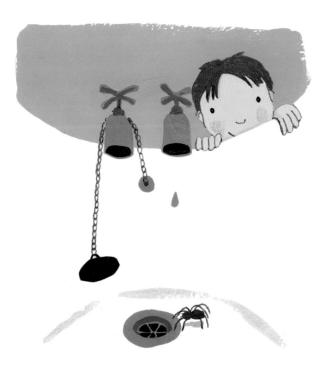

Contents

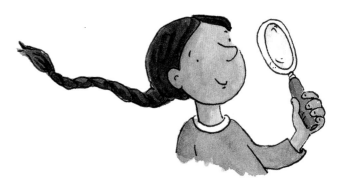

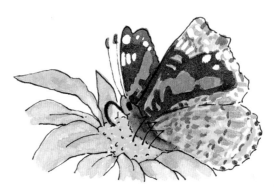

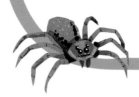